MEDICAL EDUCAT

MEDICAL EDUCATION IN EAST ASIA
Past and Future

Edited by Lincoln C. Chen,
Michael R. Reich, and Jennifer Ryan

Indiana University Press

Bloomington and Indianapolis

This book is a publication of

Indiana University Press
Office of Scholarly Publishing
Herman B Wells Library 350
1320 East 10th Street
Bloomington, Indiana 47405 USA

iupress.indiana.edu

© 2017 by Indiana University Press

All rights reserved

No part of this book may be reproduced or utilized in any form or by any means, electronic or mechanical, including photocopying and recording, or by any information storage and retrieval system, without permission in writing from the publisher. The Association of American University Presses' Resolution on Permissions constitutes the only exception to this prohibition.

♾ The paper used in this publication meets the minimum requirements of the American National Standard for Information Sciences—Permanence of Paper for Printed Library Materials, ANSI Z39.48–1992.

Manufactured in the United States of America

Library of Congress Cataloging-in-Publication Data

Names: Chen, Lincoln C., editor. | Reich, Michael, 1950- editor. | Ryan, Jennifer, 1980- editor.
Title: Medical education in East Asia : past and future / edited by Lincoln C. Chen, Michael R. Reich, and Jennifer Ryan.
Description: Bloomington and Indianapolis : Indiana University Press, [2017] | Includes bibliographical references and index.
Identifiers: LCCN 2016045752 (print) | LCCN 2016051568 (ebook) (print) | LCCN 2016051568 (ebook) | ISBN 9780253024787 (cloth : alk. paper) | ISBN 9780253024923 (pbk. : alk. paper) | ISBN 9780253025104 (ebook)
Subjects: LCSH: Medical education—East Asia. | Medical education—International cooperation—East Asia.
Classification: LCC R834 .M42 2017 (print) | LCC R834 (ebook) | DDC 610.71095—dc23
LC record available at https://lccn.loc.gov/2016045752

ISBN 978-0-253-02478-7 (cloth)
ISBN 978-0-253-02492-3 (pbk.)
ISBN 978-0-253-02510-4 (e-bk.)

1 2 3 4 5   22 21 20 19 18 17

Contents

Foreword: Bong-Min Yang, Keizo Takemi, and Yang Ke — vii
Preface: Mary Brown Bullock — ix
Acknowledgments — xiii

Part I. Overview and US-Asia Engagement — 1

History and Development of Medical Education in East Asia: An Overview
Lincoln C. Chen, Michael R. Reich, and Jennifer Ryan — 3

1. The China Medical Board in East Asia, 1950–2000
   Jennifer Ryan and Mary Brown Bullock — 21

2. American Medical Education and US Engagement in East Asia, 1950–1970
   Jesse B. Bump and Paul J. Cruickshank — 38

Part II. Country Cases: China, Japan, and South Korea — 59

3. Medical Education in Contemporary Mainland China
   Daqing Zhang — 61

4. Mission and Modernity: The History and Development of Medical Education in Taiwan
   Ming-Jung Ho, Kevin Shaw, Julie Shih, and Yu-Ting Chiu — 84

5. A Brief History of Medical Education in Hong Kong
   Gabriel M. Leung and N. G. (Niv) Patil — 112

6. The Roots of Modern Japanese Medical Education
   Kenichi Ohmi — 130

7. Western Influences on Health Science Education in Korea: Medical, Nursing, and Public Health Education
   OkRyun Moon — 158

Part III. Future Challenges   185

8 Burden of Disease: Implications for Medical Education in East Asia
Stuart Gilmour, Yusuke Tsugawa, and Kenji Shibuya   187

Contributors   209
Index   215

Foreword

Bong-Min Yang, Keizo Takemi, and Yang Ke

ANY ASSESSMENT OF contemporary medicine in East Asia must first recognize the extraordinary gains countries in the region—China, Japan, and South Korea—have achieved in extending life expectancy over the course of the past century. Our April 2014 conference on *Medical Education in East Asia: Past and Future*, celebrated the one hundredth anniversary of the China Medical Board (CMB). The sixty scholars, academics, and participants rightfully took pride in markers of success: average life expectancy of eighty-four years in Japan, eighty in South Korea, and seventy-five in China. East Asia is indisputably among the healthiest societies in the world—a triumph for a region shaped by war, political upheaval, and poverty in the twentieth century.

Many factors contribute to this success. Undeniable are the roles of political stability and economic growth, especially of the past half-century. The diffusion of modern medical sciences, professional practice, and national health systems is another major driver. The growth and development of the medical education systems in each of our countries have been profound and dramatic. Today, China, Japan, and South Korea have fairly advanced medical educational systems to produce the health professionals required for sound national health systems. All three countries are engaged in global discussions on the best means to enhance the training of twenty-first-century health professionals.

Our conference certainly provided a unique opportunity for South Korea, Japan, and China to look back on each other's medical education development during last five decades. Through the conference, all three commonly came to realize and appreciate the invaluable inputs that CMB provided in the beginning stage of development, particularly in terms of manpower training, educational materials, and even buildings for education and libraries. This conference also enabled us to look ahead, and consider what kind of contributions these three countries could offer to regional and global health.

Conference presenters took stock of conditions in the early twentieth century and then traced the evolution of medical education in Greater China, Japan, and Korea over the course of a dynamic century. The papers in this volume apply three lenses to this study: each jurisdiction's changing domestic social structures and political regimes; the nature of East Asian relationships; and the flow of Western influences, carried through the work of medical missionaries, the reforms ushered in by the Flexner Report, Cold War foreign policies, and philanthropic grant-making. While variations in organization and design are marked, the medical curriculums in all three countries clearly converge on the modern medical sciences as the most powerful means to advance the health of our peoples.

Broadening the avenue for collaboration in health in East Asia seems to be a natural step—given our shared interests in extending health gains, reducing inequities in access to care, and taking leadership roles in global health—and one that could send important signals in a region where political tensions have not abated. Sharing information in the ways this conference did, along with joint activities and other forms of cooperation in the medical education field, can ultimately benefit the health of all peoples in the region. That is a worthy goal transcending our national borders, one that is shared by us and all participants as we look forward to the next century.

Preface

Mary Brown Bullock

As it celebrated its one hundredth anniversary in 2014, the China Medical Board (CMB) sought a better understanding of the evolution of medicine and health in the Asian countries in which it had been active. After operating in China from 1914 until 1951, this American foundation turned its attention to the rest of Asia when political conditions precluded further engagement there. This volume focuses on the evolution of medical education and the role of CMB in East Asia from 1951 until 1980.

CMB engaged its Asian partners in a series of centennial celebrations and academic reviews including conferences in Bangkok, New York, Beijing, and Seoul, as well as a series of academic publications. Three volumes have been published to date: *Philanthropy for Health in China*, *Medical Transitions in Twentieth Century China*, and *Histories of Health in Southeast Asia*. This fourth volume, *Medical Education in East Asia*, emerged from papers presented at the Seoul conference, which explored a little studied topic: the evolution of China Medical Board policies and medical education and health in East Asia. CMB is grateful to the scholars who undertook new research, not only leading to deeper understanding of medical education in each country but also highlighting the many comparative themes.

The period covered begins in the early 1950s, when East Asia was flat on its back with its population decimated by war, division, political uncertainty, and desperate poverty. This was the health context to which the China Medical Board turned from China, beginning philanthropic work in Japan, Korea and Taiwan. The chapters that follow both chronicle the evolution of CMB's policies and provide country-specific case studies that illustrate the extraordinary growth and success of Asian medical education.

We must remember the challenging situation in East Asia in the 1950s. The daughter of missionaries, I lived in Japan and Korea during that period. In Tokyo, I lived in a city that still looked and felt bombed over. In Osaka, I saw my uncle struggle to organize a hospital that would care for the needy and infirm. Just after the Korean armistice, my family and I arrived in Guangju, Korea, a provincial capital of makeshift houses and hordes of beggars. I watched my father's efforts to rebuild a tuberculosis hospital while hundreds of patients waited to be treated.

Nothing I saw then—of course, I was just a little girl—would have prepared me for the transformation of economic and health conditions in East Asia that has occurred in the subsequent sixty years. What an extraordinary transformation! Economic indicators in East Asia are among the highest in the world. Medical education, whether three-year, five-year, six-year, or eight-year programs, surely played a pivotal role.

As we keep this success story in mind, we can ask the question: what are the various reasons health has improved so significantly? In several of the chapters, there are pleas to understand the historical and cultural factors behind modern medicine in Asia today. It is here that we will most likely discover the historically and culturally unique reasons for the generally healthy societies that populate East Asia today.

Another theme is the varying international inputs from both missionary and secular sources. Missionaries began as healers, and their primary legacy is the hospital, not the medical college, although some of East Asia's key medical schools had their origins in missionary work. This missionary legacy is not well-known, but it is well-chronicled in these pages. Severance Hospital in Seoul is a prime example of health care work that was started by missionaries and supplemented at a later time by organizations such as the China Medical Board. Certainly, the intersection between missionary medicine and modern medicine is one in which the CMB played a role in all of these countries.

Remembering the extraordinarily depleted Asian resources after World War II also sheds light on the rationale for various CMB policies. As the economies improved, it shifted from providing supplies and buildings to an emphasis on training faculty and building institutions. As East Asian economic medical institutions matured, CMB gradually withdrew its support to focus more on Southeast Asia, and after 1980, on returning to China. Perhaps one of its most important contributions was providing 784 fellowships for Asian medical personnel to study in the United States from 1951 to 1973.

Another key CMB policy was not to focus on one institution, as it had in China, but rather to contribute to a variety of institutions in each country. Growing Asian nationalism suggested that CMB should not attempt to dominate a single institution but, rather, identify itself with contributions to a variety of health institutions. We must also remember that CMB's Asian strategy was closely linked to the American political agenda of the post-World War II period: to help rebuild Asia and to try to tie Asian intellectuals more closely to the United States.

The Seoul workshop in March 2014 brought participants from countries that had been former colonies of Japan, Korea, and Taiwan. It also occurred at a time when political tensions between several of these countries were particularly high. This workshop may have been the first such convocation of representatives from medical universities in Japan, Korea, China, Hong Kong, and Taiwan. Some of the participants in the lively and civil dialogue were either CMB fellows themselves or trained by CMB fellows.

The China Medical Board has been privileged to play a role in this region for one hundred years. Informed by the past and looking to its next century, it anticipates an ongoing partnership with medical institutions throughout Asia.

Acknowledgments

THIS VOLUME HAD its genesis in a celebratory workshop on *Medical Education in East Asia: Past and Future*, held April 11–12, 2014, in Seoul, South Korea. The conference was part of a series of events related to the China Medical Board's centennial celebration in 2014, designed to bring new perspectives on the development of health, education, and philanthropy in Asia to wider audiences.

Many hands have helped to shape this volume, beginning with our conference co-hosts in Seoul, Seoul National University School of Public Health and Yonsei University College of Medicine. The Korean host committee was organized by Professors Bong-Min Yang and Joo-Heon Yoon, and colleagues from Korean schools who had received CMB funding during the past century, including the College of Medicine of Seoul National University, Yonsei University, Ewha Womans University, Kyung-pook National University, Chon-nam National University, and the College of Health Sciences of Korea University. Their hospitality created a warm and collegial environment, one in which our participants from Japan, Korea, China, Hong Kong, and Taiwan could share their respective histories of medical education.

We are grateful to all our conference participants, over seventy people in all—workshop paper authors; leading educators and scholars from CMB-supported medical universities in East Asia; CMB trustees Mary Brown Bullock, Tom Inui, Wendy O'Neill, and Jeffrey Williams; and Sudhir Anand of the University of Oxford—who generously shared their time and expertise. The quality of exchange among them persuaded us that these ideas should be shared more broadly, and the paper authors graciously agreed to contribute additional hours to transform their conference presentations into chapters for this volume.

Workshop logistics in Seoul were graciously handled by Eugene Kim and Ji-hyun Kim of Seoul National University. On the editorial front, we were ably assisted by Joshua Bocher, Philip Gant, and Anne Phelan, who contributed their many talents—including research, writing, and knowledge of Korean and Chinese languages—to help us prepare the final manuscript for publication.

MEDICAL EDUCATION IN EAST ASIA

PART I
OVERVIEW AND US-ASIA ENGAGEMENT

History and Development of Medical Education in East Asia: An Overview

Lincoln C. Chen, Michael R. Reich, and Jennifer Ryan

Introduction

This book explores the history and development of medical education in East Asia—China, Hong Kong, Taiwan, Japan, and South Korea—reaching back to the nineteenth century, passing through the tangles of modernization in the twentieth century, and arriving at the gates of the present in the twenty-first century. All of these countries can take pride in their spectacular health achievements—most notably, their citizens enjoy some of the longest life spans in the world—and the recent economic advances, political stability, and positive social determinants of health (like housing, basic diet, and nutrition) that helped make them possible. Success is also due, at least in part, to the development of sophisticated systems for the education of their health professionals, and so this unique volume examines the complex linkages within East Asia, the impact of international events and intellectual influences, and the domestic dynamics that shaped the medical education infrastructure in the countries in the region.

This book brings together papers the China Medical Board (CMB) commissioned for the workshop "Medical Education in East Asia: Past and Future," conducted on April 11–12, 2014, in Seoul, Korea, in celebration of CMB's centenary. That workshop, as well as events in Bangkok, New York, and Beijing, reflected CMB's intention to observe its centenary by sharing knowledge of medicine, medical education, and philanthropy in China and Asia with a wider audience. A total of seventy medical historians and educators from Korea, Japan, and Greater China attended the workshop, joined by CMB representatives and international scholars. The workshop materials are supplemented by chapters summarizing the presentations and panel discussions on twentieth-century American governmental and philanthropic influences on medical education in East Asia and twenty-first-century challenges of disease transitions there. This volume focuses on the education of physicians for clinical medicine and considers the education of professionals for public health, along with the education of health-related professionals, including nurses, dentists, pharmacists, and allied health professionals.

The essays in this book fit into the growing global attention to the health workforce, exemplified by the Commission on the Education of Health Professionals for the Twenty-First Century (Frenk et al. 2010; Hou et al. 2014). One review article of the commission's work published the year of the workshop (Crisp and Chen 2014) identified five forces shaping the global supply of health professionals: the demographic and epidemiological transitions, better education and information for patients, the revolution in biosciences and information technology, the influence of market forces, and values for social justice and human rights. The article also identified four themes in the "frontier" of education reform for health professionals: competency-based skills, changing roles of health workers, the growing importance of teamwork in health care, and innovations in learning (such as MOOCs). These four themes all appear in the chapters in this book. In addition, this book identifies another striking theme: the role of political forces—both across nations and within nations—in transforming the educational systems for health professionals.

Key Questions

The chapters in this book address core questions that arise in examining the development of medical education systems. What are the structures and functions of the medical education system in each country? What are their similarities and differences? How have the systems developed over the course of the past century, and what factors shaped their different developmental paths? How does the institutional design of medical education relate to instructional design? How have East Asia's medical education systems contributed to the region's health achievements? Answering these questions is important for the following reasons.

First, the education of health professionals constitutes a critical link between scientific knowledge and good health. Attaining good health is closely related to the production, application, and reproduction of health knowledge, which provides the tools (for example, drugs and vaccines), informs the service delivery systems (through policies and management), and educates people on health-seeking behavior. Medical universities constitute the organizational hub of knowledge for health. Through medical education, individuals are transformed into the doctors, nurses, and allied health professionals who become the human engine of health care systems, trained to drive a labor-intensive health care delivery industry. Additionally, by producing and nurturing biomedical scientists, medical universities contribute to the discovery of new knowledge. The medical education system is also responsible for the inter-generational transmission of knowledge, as senior faculty teach the students and researchers of the next generation.

Second, medical education is shaped by both instructional design and institutional design. The famous Flexner Report of 1910 revolutionized medical education by transforming the content of what is taught (science-based curriculum) and changing the location where teaching occurs (university bases with affiliated teaching hospitals). Most studies of medical education concentrate on instructional content, curriculum, and pedagogy—in short, what is learned and how it is taught. Some studies of medical education also analyze institutional design—that is, the organization of where education takes place—as they examine schools according to number, distribution, and types of professionals, organizational governance and financing, academic and professional accreditation, and policies to strengthen faculty capabilities. Yet, few studies analyze how institutional design influences, enables, and constrains instructional design—themes addressed by this volume's country studies.

This book emphasizes that understanding educational organizations is fundamental to creating effective systems that advance knowledge for producing good health. This is especially relevant for East Asian countries. These countries are undergoing profound and rapid demographic and epidemiologic transitions of aging, disability, and noncommunicable diseases (NCDs) and will need stronger, better educated, and more appropriate health professionals to promote good health, prevent disease, and treat illness. In this book, we seek to understand how the medical education systems in East Asia have contributed to the extraordinary health achievements of the recent past and what challenges they must address as they face the health problems of the twenty-first century. There are important lessons here for East Asia and for other countries around the world.

Health Indicators and Medical Education

Table 0.1 provides summary indicators of health development and medical education in the three East Asian countries. China is shown according to its territories: mainland China, Taiwan, and Hong Kong. Korea refers to the Republic of Korea on the southern portion of the peninsula. See Figure 0.1 for a map of East Asia.

The people of East Asia constitute more than a fifth of the world's population. Mainland China's population size of 1.3 billion is vast in comparison to Taiwan (23 million) and Hong Kong (7 million), ten-fold that of Japan (127 million), and twenty-five times that of South Korea (50 million). The region is an economic powerhouse. The economy of mainland China is today the second largest in the world—although its per capita gross domestic product (GDP) is one-third of Taiwan's, one-sixth of Hong Kong's, one-eighth of Japan's, and one-fourth of Korea's—and Japan has the third largest economy.

As a group, and viewed from a global perspective, these countries perform extremely well in their health achievements. Average life spans in Japan and Korea are among the highest in the world (eighty-seven years for Japanese

Table 0.1. Summary Indicators for China, Japan, and South Korea in 2012.

	China			Japan	South Korea	World
	Mainland	Taiwan	Hong Kong			
Population (millions)	1,355.00	23.1	7.2	127.3	50.2	7,046
GDP						
GDP/capita (US$)	6,100	18,300	36,700	46,500	24,400	10,172
GDP (US$, billions)	8,300		260	5,900	1,200.00	71,670
Health						
Life expectancy	76	78	83	85	81	71
Health expenditures % GDP	5.4	6.6	5.1	10.1	7.5	10.2
Public expenditures % GDP	56	58	49	82	55	60
Doctor Workforce						
Total number	1,900,000	39,186	13,203	293,391	105,009	10,569,000
Per 1,000 population	1.4	1.6	1.9	2.3	2.1	1.5
Nurse-doctor ratio	1.00	1.5	3.8	1.8	2.4	
Medical schools (number)						
Medical schools	268	12	2	81	52	2,420
Annual medical graduates	144,000	1,300	400	7,500	4,100	400,000
Curriculum (number of years)						
Total years	5 (3, 8)	6	5, 6	6	4+4	
Basic sciences	2	2	2	2	2	
Clinical sciences	2	2	2	2	1	
Practice training	1	2(+2)	1, 2	2	1	
Degrees offered	BachMed	MD	MBBS	MD	MD	

Sources: Data from World Bank 2015, Organisation for Economic Co-Operation and Development 2015, World Directory of Medical Schools 2015, Lai 2012, and the Ministry of Education of the People's Republic of China.

women), and these achievements are mirrored in Taiwan and Hong Kong. While somewhat behind, mainland China's life expectancy has accelerated in the past half century, approaching levels of other industrialized countries. In terms of health financing, Japan's 10 percent of GDP for health expenditures is about the world average, with Korea at 7.5 percent and all three territories of China at 5.1–6.6 percent. Public spending by the government overwhelmingly dominates in

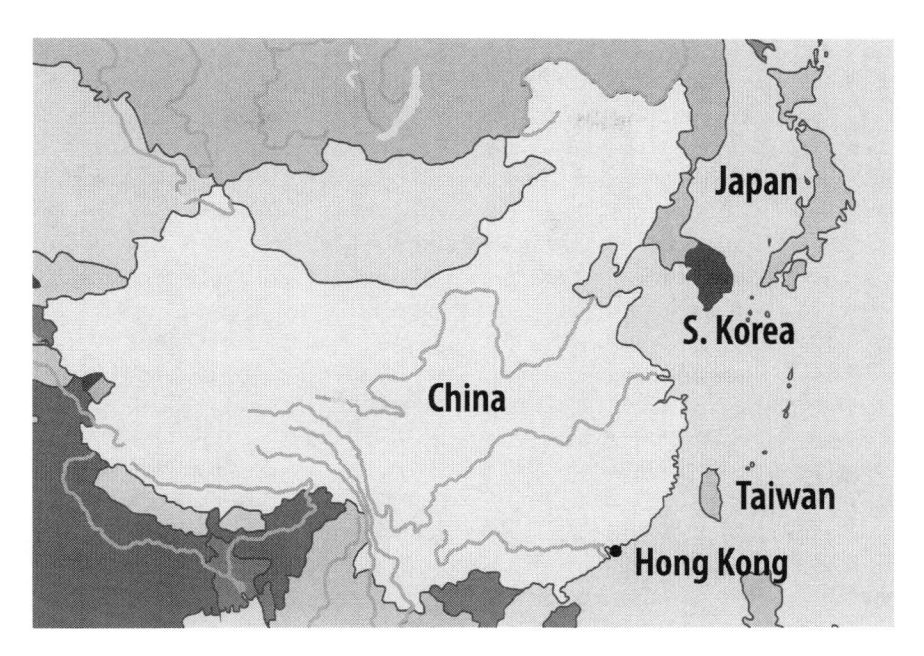

Fig. 0.1 Map of East Asia.

Japan, but it is roughly about half of total expenditures in Korea and the three Chinese territories.

The medical workforces, schools, and graduates in these three countries show both similarities and differences. China has 1.9 million doctors, or about one out of five doctors in the world, in comparison to Japan's 293,000 doctors and South Korea's 105,000 doctors. Yet, China's density of 1.4 doctors per 1,000 population is slightly lower than Taiwan and Hong Kong and significantly lower than the density of coverage found in Japan and Korea. It is noteworthy that China's about one-to-one nurse-to-doctor ratio is lower than the other countries and territories.

Mainland China has 268 medical schools, in comparison to twelve in Taiwan and two in Hong Kong, eighty-one in Japan, and fifty-two in South Korea. The numbers of annual graduates show significant differences, with graduating class sizes in mainland China vastly larger than in the other countries and territories. Whereas graduating classes in mainland China average about 537 students per cohort per school, the graduating class sizes are much smaller in Taiwan (108), Hong Kong (210), Japan (92), and South Korea (79).

Throughout East Asia, modern health professionals have been codified into distinctive professions—doctors, nurses, pharmacists, and others—following a universal pattern. In all three countries, six to eight years of post–high school education are required to produce a professional, moving from basic sciences to clinical sciences to practical training. But each country and territory also has distinctive aspects. Mainland China has several different study durations in order to meet the needs of a vast and diverse population. Its standard degree program for physicians leading to bachelors of medicine takes five years after high school, but it also has schools that offer simpler three-year and more advanced eight-year degree programs. Taiwan, Hong Kong, and Japan offer training programs of about six years duration. South Korea recently changed from the six-year duration to the American model of 4+4 years, admitting medical students after undergraduate university studies. All of the programs are designed to move students from the basic sciences to the clinical sciences and then to practical training. All of the countries and territories have professional certification validated by national examination. There is, of courses, much variability in these curricular flows—for example, in such key aspects as early exposure to patient care, education in the humanities and social sciences, and how professionalism is inculcated. Graduating degrees are mostly MDs, but bachelor and master of medicine degrees are also conferred.

Historical Paths

Over the centuries, medical education and clinical practice evolved differently in each country, but it is important to underscore the literary culture of Chinese-language characters shared among China, Japan, and Korea and related social values in the Confucian tradition. This facilitated the cultural exchange of texts, religion, and science in East Asia, including Chinese medical theory. Chinese medicine (known in the West as Traditional Chinese Medicine, or TCM) has distinctive theories backed by medicinal treatments, including acupuncture, and the use of *material medica*, its pharmacopoeia of various plants, minerals, and animals (which has led to some highly successful modern drugs, like artemisinin for treating malaria). In premodern times, before the establishment of Western-style universities, the knowledge and practice of Chinese medicine was tested through trial and error and passed down through the generations from master to disciple or from father to son.

Western science traveled to East Asia during the sixteenth century with Christian missionaries. Encounters with Western medical knowledge expanded with missionary movements of the nineteenth century, which included church-sponsored clinics and hospitals. In the eighteenth century, Japan translated medical texts of Dutch physicians, and by 1861, it opened its first Western-style hospital. Korea's first Western hospital, Jejungwon in Seoul, opened in 1885. In Taiwan, the Dutch and Spanish first brought Western medicine in the early seventeenth century, and they were followed by medical missionaries. By the mid- to late-nineteenth century, missionary-sponsored schools and hospitals were functioning in many cities across China, including the Medical Missionary Hospital of Hong Kong, which opened its doors in 1843. The combination of medical missionaries and medical philanthropy resulted in the establishment of the Peking Union Medical College in Beijing by the Rockefeller Foundation in 1917 (Bullock 1980).

In the twentieth century, the social and political transformations of East Asian countries had dramatic impacts on the national development of medical education and the role of different Western models. For example, through a series of wars and conflicts in the first half of the century, China experienced the collapse of the Qing Dynasty, the establishment of the Republic of China in 1912, and the founding of the People's Republic of China in 1949. During the Republican period, China studied foreign models of medicine from Japan, Europe, and the United States. This changed, however, in the second half of the twentieth century, when China took the Soviet-style path of medicine with its early socialist health campaigns (Gao 2014). Later, medical education in China was twice radically altered and reconstructed, with the Cultural Revolution and then again when the country opened its economy to the global market. Japan, after the Meiji Restoration in 1868, adopted a German-Japanese model of medical education and, in the early twentieth century, exported that model to its colonies of Korea and Taiwan. After World War II, Japan was compelled by the US occupation to reform its medical education system along American lines. At the same time, South Korea achieved independence and Taiwan became the Republic of China, and both were influenced by the US model of medical education and postwar US aid. Hong Kong, on the other hand, as a crown colony of the United Kingdom until its return to China in 1997, followed a British system of medical education. These historical landmarks are keys for understanding the major shifts of the medical education in the three countries.

This brief comparison shows the striking influences of the German, American, British, and Soviet models of medical education in East Asia. All of these national systems of medical education developed out of the scientific revolution and the rapid development of modern medicine in the second half of the nineteenth century. Previously, medical training had not been regularized and standardized, and various forms of Western medicine—such as humorism, Galenic medicine, surgery, and folk remedies—had been commonly practiced for centuries. Sharing a common foundation in Western science, the newly emerging systems of medical education were introduced into East Asia and came into interaction with that region's own set of varied medical practices.

These four national models of medical education each had distinctive features. The German system, with its authority grounded in the modern scientific discoveries of the nineteenth century, aimed to produce physician-scientists through competitive admission of students with undergraduate degrees to enter an elite profession, training in scientific investigation in laboratories, and clinical training in a university hospital. German medical schools were closely associated with universities, sometimes following a "Prussian officer" model with hierarchical power exercised by the heads of medical departments. The US system, powerfully shaped by the path-breaking 1910 Flexner Report, also aimed to produce physician-scientists with science-based training in problem solving from universities and practice-based training at teaching hospitals. Admission to American medical schools required an undergraduate degree. The UK system, on the other hand, directly admitted high school graduates to medical schools. But medical education in the United Kingdom was still linked with universities and the profession was increasingly standardized (under the influence of Flexner's report) to reform its apprenticeship system and reduce fragmentation of the profession. The Soviet system, also based in Western scientific methods, was ideologically bound (e.g., Marxist dialectical materialism and "Lysenko" theory), with medical education and health care rigidly controlled under centralized direction. Perhaps the biggest difference among these national models of medical education is that Soviet training institutions were "free-standing" health training institutes under the control of the ministry of health, whereas the German, United States, and British models placed medical education within universities.

China's medical education system has only recently changed from the Soviet to the Anglo-American model, with an important aspect being the shift of authority and control from the Ministry of Health to the Ministry of Education. Taiwan and Hong Kong have maintained their own systems—Taiwan since the Republic of China was established and Hong Kong despite its return from the United Kingdom to China. Japan maintains a mixture of a new Anglo-American system built on top of German-Japanese traditions, whereas Korea has, since independence, built a mostly Anglo-American model of education.

Medical Education in East Asia

This book examines the historical development of medical education in East Asia in three sections. Part I provides a review of the China Medical Board's activities in Asia in the second half of the twentieth century and an analysis of how American medicine evolved and engaged with East Asia, with a focus on the mid-twentieth century. Part II explores and explains the development of medical education in mainland China, Taiwan, Hong Kong, Japan, and South Korea, with separate chapters on each. Finally, part III presents the demographic and epidemiologic transitions in East Asia and their implications for future medical education systems.

CMB was instrumental in the twentieth-century development of medical education, as shown by Mary Brown Bullock and Jennifer Ryan in chapter 1. They demonstrate that CMB supported medical education not only in China, as its name suggests, but in a total of seventeen countries throughout East Asia. In their presentation of CMB's institutional history, Bullock and Ryan describe how it expanded its mission after PUMC was nationalized in 1949, when the American foundation was forced to pull out of the newly established People's Republic of China. Turning this exodus into an opportunity, the foundation changed direction and strategy, deciding to make investments in other countries where its philanthropic mission would serve the needs of the "Far East," as the region was then known. Over the next thirty years, CMB had significant impacts throughout East Asia (outside China), funding strategic projects that met countries' specific needs in medical education. The foundation funded reconstruction projects, granted institutional matching endowment funds, and supported hundreds of individuals in travel fellowships and exchange programs. It also made other contributions to the development of medical education in Asia, including small but singular achievements such as building and stocking the first and only medical library in the Philippines and translating the first textbooks on nursing into Chinese.

In chapter 2, Jesse B. Bump and Paul J. Cruickshank present the evolution of medical education in the United States, starting with an overview of the 1910 Flexner Report and its influence. The Flexner Report provided the foundation for reforming the US medical education system and for the promotion of America's post–World War II emphasis on biomedical research. Bump and Cruickshank highlight how federal funding through the National Institutes of Health (NIH) to universities during the Cold War catapulted medical research and scientific discovery into the forefront of US medical education. Subsequently, partly in reaction to this shift, there emerged a renewed interest in clinical care centered in teaching hospitals. This chapter also analyzes how US foreign policy promoted medical research in East Asia. For example, the NIH opened a Pacific office in Tokyo in 1962 in order to advance biomedical research in the region. The analysis in this chapter found some tension between the scientific goals of the NIH and the political goals of the US government in the Cold War period. However, by the end of the twentieth century, the influence of scientific medicine dominated medical education across East Asia, a region where traditional medicine had reigned for centuries. The following chapters explore how this happened in the different countries of East Asia.

In chapter 3, Daqing Zhang traces the development of medical education in mainland China, focusing on the post-1949 period. He specifically examines how severe political tides affected both the instructional and the institutional design of medical colleges. He shows how medical education experienced radical transformations in the second half of the twentieth century: from the influence of central planning and Soviet-style education, to the complete disruption of higher education during the Cultural Revolution, and (under current pressure) to the production of a medical workforce for nationwide health care reforms. Medical education in China has thus grappled with profound tensions: politics versus medicine, tradition versus modernity, and elite-oriented versus popular-oriented goals. These tensions include, among other issues, the complex questions of where TCM fits in contemporary society and medical education and how to remedy the erosion of the doctor-patient relationship and trust, which has resulted in serious patient-on-doctor violence in health care facilities throughout China.

In chapter 4, Ming-Jung Ho and colleagues show how medical education has been a vehicle for modernization on Taiwan. They examine the intersection of local people and international political forces, including Western colonization and missionaries, Qing rule and defeat, Japanese colonialism, the emergence of the Republic of China, and US aid and influence. The synthesis of the different pressures on medical education and the question of how to make medical education "globally viable and locally coherent" have been major challenges for Taiwan. Ho and her associates explain how today's complex system has evolved to combine traditional medicine licensure and Confucian values within a system dominated by Western medicine. For at least the past sixty years, institutional design and quality of medical school graduates have been pressing issues in Taiwan. While much progress has been made, the medical school reforms in 2013 reflect continued concerns about clinical competencies not being met, shortages of certain types of doctors, and challenges to medical professionalism. Taiwan is also seeking to develop a medical curriculum that respects local cultural values, including, for example, the role of a Confucian perspective in both personal and professional affairs.

As it did in Taiwan and the mainland, Western medicine entered Hong Kong through missionaries and against the backdrop of Chinese medicine. In chapter 5, Gabriel Leung and N. G. Patel recount the primarily British roots of modern Western medical education in Hong Kong. Hong Kong became a British colony in 1841, after the First Opium War, as a result of the Treaty of Nanking. For almost a century, the Hong Kong College of Medicine, founded in 1877, was the only medical school in Hong Kong, until a second medical school was established in 1974 in order to meet the growing demand for health care professionals. Hong Kong remained a British colony until its repatriation to China in 1997, and as a result, its health care system and medical education have closely followed the British model. Yet today, despite Hong Kong's international outlook, the medical economy is "relatively closed." For example, it is difficult for physicians not educated in a Hong Kong medical school to practice medicine there. On the other hand, Leung and Patil argue in this chapter that the Hong Kong Academy of Medicine and its constituent medical schools are uniquely positioned culturally and geographically to serve as a link between Hong Kong and mainland China for regional development and cooperation and for developing a "new model of integrative medicine" that combines Western methods with traditional Chinese medical practice. The extent to which Hong Kong can fulfill that promise into the future—as the arbiter between East and West—remains to be seen.

In chapter 6, on the evolution of medical education in Japan, Kenichi Ohmi focuses on the cultural and institutional history of medical training in that country. The chapter describes how Western medicine came to replace traditional medicine after the Meiji Restoration in 1868 and Japan's opening to the outside world. Ohmi notes that status differentials persisting from Japan's feudal society during the Edo period translated into hierarchical medical institutions that produced samurai doctors and lower status practitioners. He also explores how current domestic challenges for medical education are rooted in this historical context. For example, during the Edo period, the Dutch introduced Western medicine (specifically the German system of medical education), as Prussian military medicine was more compatible with samurai customs. The Japanese then took this system of medical education to colonial Korea and Taiwan in the early twentieth century. But even as the Japanese instituted Flexnerian reforms based on the American model of medical education after World War II, including the insertion of clinical training into the curriculum in 1968, some traditional cultural patterns have continued to exert powerful influence. Ohmi argues, for example, that an overemphasis on passing the National Examination and a lack of focus on liberal arts in medical education have both been detrimental to composition of the health care workforce produced by the medical education system.

Next, in chapter 7, OkRyun Moon examines Korea's medical education system, with particular attention to domestic challenges and international linkages. He first describes the external forces in the seventeenth to nineteenth centuries that brought Western medicine to Korea during the Joseon dynasty. Medicine in Korea had long developed under the influence of TCM until Japanese traders introduced Western medicine. Western missionaries then expanded the role of Western medicine when they opened the first Western hospital in 1885 and the first Western medical school in 1899. In the early twentieth century, medical education in Korea came under the control of Japanese colonial rule. In the postwar shift, the newly established Republic of Korea was heavily influenced by the US system of medical education, adopting its textbooks and clinical programs, as well as accreditation and best practices. It has been a century of change for medical education in Korea, including, more recently, Korea's sharing in a global move toward patient-centered care, emphasis on continuing education, and role in international health aid. The results of these developments, including strategies for domestic challenges and prospects for the future, are among the issues considered in this chapter.

The book's third section provides a concluding, eighth chapter by Kenji Shibuya and colleagues that presents a comparative analysis of disease burden and risk factors in the three East Asian countries—China, Japan, and South

Korea. Using data analysis from the 2010 Global Burden of Disease (GBD) study, they examine the growing burden of NCDs in the region, highlighting both commonalities and differences in population health. As is well known, the East Asia region has experienced dramatic and rapid health gains since the mid-twentieth century, reflected in significant mortality reductions for all age groups (with Japan's life expectancy among the highest in the world). As a result, many disease burden and risk factors are now shared by these countries, including stroke, cancer, smoking, dietary risks, and high blood pressure. But this chapter's analysis also reveals important differences: China has increased levels of air pollution and infectious diseases, whereas Japan has more obesity and a rapidly aging population. Shibuya and his associates identify lessons learned from the experiences of these countries, such as public health interventions targeted at reducing disease and the ways national burden of disease analysis can be used for national policy development. The chapter concludes with a discussion of the need for medical education to keep pace with epidemiological transitions and the implications for the future of health systems in East Asia in an interconnected world.

Cross-Cutting Themes in Medical Education

Three cross-cutting themes in medical education emerge from the chapters in this book: first, the role of international political processes in shaping medical education; second, the role of domestic political processes in shaping that education; and third, the common substantive challenges now confronting all medical education systems in East Asia. These common challenges include tensions between tradition and modernity, conflicts between an elite-orientation and a popular-orientation, and institutional and instructional design strategies.

Influence of International Politics

The history of medical education in East Asia shows how major issues of system design have been dramatically swayed by international political events, including war, colonialism, independence, trade, and missionaries. The changes often resulted in discarding old patterns and adopting new national models. The flows across space and national boundaries have had an effect not only in East Asia, but also globally. Many of these flows have deep historical roots, including the movements of different forms of traditional medicine across the region before the introduction of Western scientific medicine.

The histories in this book show that foreign medical education policy was sometimes imposed by an outside force on a country. Three examples are colonialism by Japan (such as Japanese banning of traditional Chinese medicine in Taiwan and the building of Japanese medical schools in Taiwan and Korea), US military victory and occupation of Japan in the postwar period (which emphasized the US medical education system and imposed its standards on Japan), and British colonial imposition of its medical education system on Hong Kong (creating the only British medical education model in the region).

On the other hand, sometimes countries independently adopted foreign medical education policy from the outside. This pattern is illustrated by Japanese adoption of German medical education as a conscious autonomous decision in the early Meiji period, mainland China's decision to adopt American and European models of medical education during the Nationalist period and then the Soviet model in the early communist period, and historical examples of Korea, Japan, and Taiwan adopting traditional Chinese medicine.

Influence of Domestic Politics

Domestic political conflicts and transitions have also shaped how the medical education systems evolved in each country studied in this book. For example, Japan's decision to ban traditional Chinese medicine was driven largely by domestic political forces. In other countries as well, decisions about medical education systems have been influenced by conflict among different visions of medical practice and different medical education institutions that embody those visions of medical practice. The decision by Chinese communists to change medical education during the Cultural Revolution period "disrupted" the training of physicians—indeed, for four years (1966–1970), all medical education "ground to a halt." Even after the higher education system was restarted, questions about what constituted "good medical education remained a controversial issue," as pointed out in chapter 3. Zhang concludes there that "the evolution of medical education in China occurred under a series of political interventions, rather than as an independent progress consisting of adaptations to the social and economic environment."

It is worth noting that domestic politics (in this case China's revolutionary politics) also shaped the China Medical Board's role in Asia. When CMB was forced out of China following the Communist Revolution of 1949, the foundation decided to seek a new role and mission to replace its single-country focus on China and its single-institution focus on Peking Union Medical College (as presented in chapter 2). But CMB did not voluntarily decide to change its focus. The result was three decades of expansion and diversification throughout Asia— first to Japan and Taiwan in 1952, next to Korea, Hong Kong, and Thailand in 1953, and ultimately to medical institutions in sixteen countries. This expansion and diversification in Asia and in themes has continued in CMB's most recent period under president Lincoln Chen (2007–present), both in China and in the rest of East Asia, with its new emphasis on supporting broader health professional education, strengthening capacity in health policy and health systems, and addressing rural health issues. In many ways, CMB has the Communist Revolution to thank for forcing it to transform itself and find new ways to relate to health in Asia—beyond China and beyond medicine.

Common Substantive Challenges

Tradition and modernity: Throughout East Asia, and indeed across the world, Western medical systems have not only achieved a foothold but have experienced tremendous growth. In these shifts, a common tension has been between tradition and modernity, although it has complementarity as well as competition. As East Asian countries sought to modernize, they sometimes licensed existing practitioners of traditional medicine without requiring them to pass examinations in Western medicine, while at other times such requirements were imposed. In some periods, such practitioners were suppressed, but in others, strategies were sought to integrate traditional medicine into the new educational systems.

In all East Asian countries today, traditional medicine coexists with Western medicine, enjoying both popular use and national support. Traditional medicine has its own schools and universities for specialized training, national licensing exams, standards for prescription medicines, and medical insurance reimbursements, as well as national associations that promote and support its teaching, clinical practice, and research, such as the Association of Korean Medicine, the Japan Society for Oriental Medicine, and the State Administration of Traditional Chinese Medicine. The resulting picture of medical education systems is one of commonality and diversity distinctive to the region. All countries have systems of medical education that are based on Western scientific medicine but integrated with local strains of traditional medical education and practice. The School of Chinese Medicine at The University of Hong Kong's Li Ka Shing Faculty of Medicine, for example, promotes interdisciplinary research on traditional medicine, while China Medical University in Taiwan offers training in both Western and Chinese medicine. At universities of Chinese medicine in mainland China, courses in Western medicine are required.

A question for the future of national health systems is how to integrate traditional medicine into modern (Western) medical education and manage the bi-directional influences between traditional systems and Western medical theory and practice. These new mixed patterns could form the core of a deeper consideration of integrative medicine within and across East Asian countries.

Elite versus popular orientation: A great tension exists in East Asian countries between an elite orientation and a popular orientation—goals of excellence, prestige, and hierarchy competing with efforts to produce health professionals for health care at the level of the larger population, especially affordable access to quality health care for the poor and disadvantaged. While China today seeks to produce world-class scientists, the aim of the earlier "barefoot doctors" movement was to bring basic health care to rural areas during the Cultural Revolution. Currently in China, elite eight-year medical schools in metropolitan Beijing and Shanghai produce specialists for urban hospital practice, while three-year schools in rural areas produce general practitioners to train and retain local primary care doctors for China's rural population. Japan adopted the "Prussian officer" system of medical education in the Edo and Meiji eras, with elite schools like Tokyo University admitting students of samurai backgrounds with high status and focusing on theory and thinking while medical practice was relegated to the lower-status professional schools.

In each country, a hierarchy exists, both explicit and implicit, within medical institutions—prestige, scientific excellence, and specialization being at the top and general practice at the bottom—with the result that factors such as salary, reputation, job security, and placement provide greater incentives for health professionals to enter certain fields rather than others. In Taiwan, for example, low reimbursement for primary care in the national health insurance system has caused a shortage of primary care physicians, while in Japan, despite a surplus of doctors nationwide, there is a shortage of doctors in rural areas. All of these countries confront distributional challenges such as how to persuade medical school graduates to practice medicine in primary and rural health care and how to align professional incentives to meet health workforce objectives. Each also faces its own complex set of issues in addressing health insurance and health systems in medical education, especially the challenges of avoiding an elite orientation that is set disproportionately over the goals of a popular orientation.

Institutional and instructional design: The chapters on individual countries in part II of this book underscore the relationship between institutional design and instructional design, two important and interdependent aspects of medical education. Institutional design significantly affects health systems, since it determines how many of what kinds of professionals will be produced for roles in national health care systems, whereas instructional design focuses on teaching and learning within the institution (i.e., the curriculum and pedagogy).

The institutional base—consisting of organizational number, distribution, type, governance, financing, accreditation, and faculty development—organizes instruction, and an educational organization must have teaching and learning to fulfill its mandate. The powerful influence of institutional design on instruction, however, is underappreciated. For example, the recent reform and expansion of medical institutions in China carries the danger of dilution of quality because student enrollment has far outstripped facilities and faculty capacity. Many innovative techniques like problem-based learning are not possible where faculty-to-student ratios are low or where interactive classroom space is not available. High-quality instructional design ensures a competent workforce, but institutional design shapes the number and kinds of professionals that will be available to drive the entire health system. For example, admissions policy determines whether rural candidates have been admitted who, thus, are more likely to consider rural service. Because professional education is a lengthy process and institutions require systematic investments, institutional design has a decade-long or even generation-long time trajectory.

Despite massive improvements in health and medical education over the twentieth century, current national medical education systems are not producing enough of the needed types of high-quality physicians to serve the populations of East Asia, and these chapters, focused on individual countries, illustrate the tension between education for researchers and education for clinicians and the tension between producing scientists and producing practitioners. Moreover, there are tensions between medical education and health care systems, including competition for use of faculty time in connection with national health programs (for example, Medicare in the United States and universal health in Taiwan, in which teachers are spending more time in clinical practice rather than in teaching students). On the curricular level, shared concerns include implementing problem-based learning and the role of social sciences and humanities in medical education, including how to address the role of "traditional" values in medical education. Across East Asia, a variety of factors—from increased patient-on-doctor violence in China and Taiwan, to students reporting a lack of confidence in clinical skills, to a focus on passing written exams over developing practical skills—demonstrate that instruction needs earlier and better clinical training in interpersonal communication skills to support the development of effective and appropriate "bedside manner." Training students in a core set of clinical competencies is central to producing "high-quality" physicians, while developing the norms and standards of medical professionalism—professional ethics in particular—is essential for registering and monitoring them in appropriate ways.

Conclusions

The quality of the health professional educational system in Greater China, Japan, and Korea will be critical for meeting emerging health challenges in the future. All are confronted by the "triple tsunami" of aging, NCDs, and disability. These societies will be comprised of the most elderly populations in the world. More than four-fifths of the causes of death are due to NCDs, and the burden of disability is growing dramatically. New and more appropriately trained health professionals will be required to grapple with these challenges and develop fresh prevention strategies, primary and home-based team care; effective management of new technologies; efficient vertical referrals in the health care system; and social, economic, and ethical behaviors for both doctors and patients. Asia will seek to devise its own solutions, no longer simply adopting Western models, as learning becomes multidirectional facilitated by global interactions. There is every expectation that China, Japan, and Korea will become innovators and pioneers in forming and reforming the systems of health professional education for the twenty-first century.

References

Bullock, Mary Brown. 1980. *An American Transplant: The Rockefeller Foundation and Peking Union Medical College.* Berkeley: University of California Press.

Crisp, Nigel, and Lincoln Chen. "Global Supply of Health Professionals." *New England Journal of Medicine* 370: 950–57.

Frenk, Julio, Lincoln Chen, Zulfiqar, A. Bhutta, Jordan Cohen, Nigel Crisp, Timothy Evans, Harvey Fineberg, et al. 2010. "Health Professionals for a New Century: Transforming Education to Strengthen Health Systems in an Interdependent World." *The Lancet* 376: 1923–58.

Gao, Xi. 2014. "Foreign Models of Medicine in Twentieth-Century China." In *Medical Transitions in Twentieth-Century China*, edited by Bridie Andrews and Mary Brown Bullock, 173–211. Bloomington: Indiana University Press.

Hou, Jianlin, Catherine Michaud, Zhihui Li, Zhe Dong, Baoshi Sun, Junhua Zhang, Depin Cao, et al. 2014. "Transformation of the Education of Health Professionals in China: Progress and Challenges." *The Lancet* 384: 819–27.

Lai, Chi-Wan. 2012. "A Critical Review of the Medical Education in Taiwan." Presented at Taiwan Medical Accreditation Council on April 22, 2012. Last accessed July 2, 2016. www.heeact.edu.tw/public/Attachment/24261893137.pdf.

Ministry of Education of the People's Republic of China. "Number of Health Professional Graduates by Major, Degree and School, 1998–2012." Unpublished.

Organization for Economic Co-Operation and Development. 2015. "OECD.Stat." Last accessed July 2, 2016. http://stats.oecd.org/index.aspx.

World Bank. 2015. "Indicators." Last accessed July 2, 2016. http://data.worldbank.org/indicator.

World Directory of Medical Schools. 2015. "World Directory of Medical Schools." https://wdoms.org.

1 The China Medical Board in East Asia, 1950–2000

Jennifer Ryan and Mary Brown Bullock

Introduction

The China Medical Board was instrumental to the twentieth-century development of medical education, not only in China, as its name would suggest, but in a total of seventeen countries outside the United States, including all of the countries in East Asia. This chapter on the institutional history of CMB describes how it expanded its mission after the Peking Union Medical College (PUMC) was nationalized and the American foundation was forced to pull out of the newly established People's Republic of China. Turning this exodus into an opportunity, the foundation made adjustments and strategic investments to maximize impact where its philanthropic mission could best serve the needs of the "Far East," as the region was known at the time. Indeed, the region was in great need of reconstruction after the damages of the wartime years. During its thirty years outside China, CMB continued to make a significant impact by funding strategic projects as it recognized specific country needs. The foundation funded reconstruction projects, granted institutional matching endowment funds, and supported hundreds of individuals with travel fellowships and exchange programs. Although they were less well-known than these long-term impact grants, CMB made other unique contributions to the development of medical education in Asia—including small but singular achievements such as building and stocking the first and only medical library in the Philippines and translating the first textbooks on nursing into Chinese.

Overview

Over the course of a century, by building medical institutions in China and neighboring Asian countries, CMB has given hundreds of millions of dollars in grants and technical support to strengthen education and research in medicine, nursing, and public health, all aimed at improving health in Asia. In the first half of the twentieth century, most of CMB's resources went toward the construction and development of PUMC to establish a world-class medical school and hospital in China. Virtually all of the premier medical universities in Asia have been funded in some way by CMB, including many schools focusing on rural health in remote regions. In its one-hundred-year history, CMB has provided US $1.5 billion to more than 118 Asian medical universities, supporting young and senior fellows and funding innovations in research and education. Innovation has been a hallmark of CMB's impact in Asia, from research innovations such as the isolation of ephedrine, the discovery of Peking Man, and the first model of rural primary health care deploying "barefoot doctors" to educational innovations like the introduction and dissemination of science-based education in universities, problem-based and standardized patient learning, global minimal educational requirements, and IT-accelerated learning.

Over the course of one hundred years, CMB—one of the earliest modern philanthropic institutions to operate in Asia—has been led by eight presidents and seventy trustees, including John D. Rockefeller III, who served on the board from 1930 to 1947. Programmatic shifts reflect changing historical circumstances, while the long tenure of CMB's leadership highlights its lasting engagements with and deep knowledge of Asia over a transformative era. The institutional history of CMB that follows has been taken largely from its annual reports and archival materials from 1914 to 2014.

The PUMC Era: 1914–1950

The more than three decades between 1914 and 1950 could be dubbed "The PUMC Era." Following the recommendations of *Medicine in China*, a report published by the China Medical Commission of the Rockefeller Foundation, CMB was launched in 1914 as the second major program of the newly established Rockefeller Foundation. The CMB was created to put the ideas of the commission into practice, specifically to manage funding and operations for the establishment of PUMC, "the cradle of modern medicine in China." Indeed, CMB spent the next three decades constructing, staffing, and developing China's premier medical school and affiliated teaching hospital until it had to pull its operations from China when PUMC was nationalized after 1949 by the newly victorious Chinese Communist government.

CMB's mission today traces its roots to the early years of the twentieth century, when breakthroughs in science were opening a new era of science-based medicine and Abraham Flexner's path-breaking report was beginning to transform modern medical education. John D. Rockefeller Sr., the richest man of his generation, was channeling his vast wealth toward philanthropic endeavors through the newly created Rockefeller Foundation, and CMB was its second and perhaps largest-ever program.

CMB's intellectual foundations and mandate for its work in China were expressed in the ninety-eight-page commission report funded by the Rockefeller Foundation. In April 1914, the members of the commission—Harry Pratt Judson,

Roger Sherman Greene, Francis Weld Peabody, and George Baldwin McKibbin—sailed to China to examine various medical schools and hospitals and report on the conditions of public health and medicine there. All in all, they surveyed seventeen medical schools and ninety-seven hospitals on their trip, which extended to eleven of China's eighteen provinces. The commission met with both government officials and those who ran the medical missionary schools. Those early decades found China at a crossroads as the collapse of the Qing Dynasty gave way to the beginning of the new Republic of China and major efforts at modernization were poised to improve the health of the country trying to shed the moniker "the sick man of Asia." The health conditions surveyed by the commission included incidences of infectious diseases such as cholera and bubonic plague, as well as tuberculosis, hookworm, and syphilis, and also assessed the state of medicine and surgery at that time, western medicine in China, and standards of medical education under missionary auspices. Through their extensive travels and observations, the commission members were convinced that the time and Chinese receptivity were ripe for the introduction of western medical teaching and practice (China Medical Commission of the Rockefeller Foundation 1914).

Recommendations included that the Rockefeller Foundation should certainly undertake medical work in China, cooperate with existing missionary institutions as far as possible, and instill the highest standards of medical instruction in English. The commission recommended that medical educational work begin in Beijing in connection with the existing Union Medical College. In 1915, the foundation purchased and assumed support of the Union Medical College, which had been founded by a group of Protestant missionaries in 1906. Construction of the physical plant took the next four years. In 1917, CMB established PUMC to expand western medicine in China, and in 1919, PUMC admitted women for nursing, becoming the first coeducational school in China. By 1921, formal dedication ceremonies were held on the campus grounds, with John D. Rockefeller Jr. declaring the intention to "make permanent on Chinese soil the best in scientific medicine that the world can offer."[1] The first meeting of the board of trustees in September 1921 was attended by fourteen members, including Rockefeller Jr.

PUMC was a first-rate biomedical research facility, and English was the language of instruction. PUMC's research departments included anatomy, chemistry, physiology, and pathology, as well as a radiology, or X-ray, department. In 1924, PUMC scientists discovered and isolated ephedrine from the Chinese herb *mahuang* (*Ephedra sinica*). Two years later, Davidson Black discovered Peking Man and conducted paleontology studies in PUMC's Department of Anatomy. PUMC quickly became the premier medical school and hospital in China, so prominent, in fact, that China's first president, Dr. Sun Yat-sen (Sun Zhongshan), also a physician of western medicine, chose to be evaluated at PUMC before he died of liver cancer in 1925. That same year, public health pioneers John Grant and C. C. Chen established and developed the first health-field station in Beijing, which was staffed by PUMC students, and then began rural health work in Ding Xian, which eventually developed into the "barefoot doctor" model.

In 1928, the CMB received its first Rockefeller Foundation endowment of $12 million to create an independent American foundation for the continuing support of PUMC. Shortly thereafter, leading Chinese philosopher and modernizer Hu Shih joined PUMC's board, becoming Chairman from 1946–1949. Throughout both the Sino-Japanese and Chinese civil wars, PUMC's dedicated staff and leadership steadfastly continued CMB's mission. During this period, led by visionaries and medical men (both Chinese and western) such as John B. Grant and Hu Shih, and others such as C. U. Lee, Roger Greene, and Henry S. Houghton, PUMC doctors and nurses cared for wounded soldiers during Japanese invasion. When PUMC was taken over during World War II, the Japanese interned Director Henry Houghton, who remained captive for four years (1942–1946).

With the outbreak of war with Japan in 1941 and the occupation of PUMC by Japanese troops, CMB redirected PUMC students it supported to continue their studies at other medical schools. PUMC reopened in 1947 with twenty-two medical and sixteen nursing students, led by C. U. Lee, its first Chinese director. Yet, the resumption of full-scale operation of the college was not possible.

With the success of the Communist Revolution in 1949, conditions began to change. The CMB planned to continue work in the People's Republic of China, but the advent of the Korean War and worsening relations between the two governments made this impossible. In January 1951, PUMC was nationalized and all funds for China were frozen by the US government. CMB, under Director Harold Loucks, withdrew from the newly formed People's Republic of China and would not return for almost thirty years. At the same time that CMB was forced to leave the mainland, PUMC graduates and former staff members who left with the Chiang Kai-shek's Nationalists joined together and formed the National Defense Medical Center in Taiwan for the training of medical students there.

By 1951, PUMC faculty and graduates had founded many key clinical specialties in China and developed innovations such as a three-tiered rural health system. The knowledge generated by PUMC helped usher in a revolution in the understanding and practice of medicine in China that catalyzed dramatic health progress, and its graduates, including Huang Jiasi and Wu Jieping, have made enduring contributions to China's health care system.

CMB Extends to East and Southeast Asia: 1951–1980

Political change in China interrupted CMB's work on the mainland for three decades and prompted CMB's extension throughout Asia in the 1950s. Since CMB could no longer continue its support of PUMC, in 1951 it began to expand its program to medical and nursing schools to the limits permitted by its charter to "the Far East and the United States of America." In a time of stress and uncertainty, CMB's board of trustees widened their field of activity, entering new geographies with a new program strategy. The year 1952 marked CMB's first grants in new territories. Support went first to Japan and Taiwan in 1952, next to Korea, Hong Kong, and Thailand in 1953, and ultimately, over the following three decades, to medical institutions in fourteen countries and regions outside the United States and China, including medical schools in the Philippines, Indonesia, Ceylon (Sri Lanka), Malaya (Malaysia), Burma (Myanmar), Singapore, and Vietnam.[2]

Table 1.1 shows the number of grantee schools and total funding in East Asia over three decades. A full listing of grantee schools from Table 1.1 can be found in the annex at the end of this chapter. Among this group, South Korea received the most funding, with $9.1 million, followed by Taiwan, Japan, and Hong Kong. It is interesting to note that, while the number of grantee schools in Japan (forty schools) far exceeded any other country, the overall level of funding to the country was much lower compared with countries with fewer number of schools (in the case of Hong Kong, only one school). This kind of differentiated grant making by the CMB board was in response to local schools' needs and strengths and changing socioeconomic conditions within the region.

During these thirty years, CMB's program outside mainland China funded a wide swath of projects as it recognized needs in specific countries. This was of particular value in light of in-country reorganization and reconstruction efforts during the postwar years. In the early days of CMB's new program in the Far East, the projects aided by its grants fell into the following four major categories: fellowships, visiting professorships, medical libraries, and equipment for laboratories. Individuals sponsored by CMB fellowships and visiting professorships crisscrossed the globe—Asian physician-teachers traveled to US institutions for educational exchanges while American professors taught as medical faculty in Asian institutions. Institutions sponsored by CMB were able to rebuild and stock libraries and equip their schools to carry out research and teaching activities.

Table 1.1. CMB East Asian Medical University Grantees, 1951–1980.

Country	Number of Schools	Total Funding (in millions)
Japan	40	3.1
South Korea	8	9.1
Taiwan	4	7.0
Hong Kong	1	2.2

Source: Norris 2003, 266–67 (Appendix I-5).

Fellowships

For over twenty years, CMB made individual fellowship grants to medical and nursing schools in the region. It considered its fellowship program for study and travel in the United States one of its most important contributions to medical education in the Far East. Study fellowships provided for one year of study, usually in the United States or occasionally in Europe, while travel fellowships would enable those with an already established scientific reputation to bring themselves up to date with developments in their field of interest. Most recipients would travel to the United States for a period of about three to six months to visit American schools and hospitals to observe their operations. During the first year of the fellowship program (1952), funds were given to thirteen medical schools for sixteen fellowships.

It was CMB's view that the fellowship program was to improve medical education in the recipient's home country, not just enhance his or her personal career. Concerned that these not contribute to "brain drain" in the medical sciences, CMB granted fellowships with the expectation that the individual was to return to his or her school after completion.

Japan, a CMB grant recipient until 1974, received the highest number of fellowships, with a total of 186, with Taiwan right behind with 185, followed by Thailand and Korea with 106 and 100, respectively. Of the total number of fellowships, study fellowships made up the bulk of the total at 78 percent, with travel fellowships at 22 percent (see Table 1.2). Support was given to various disciplines, including: clinical sciences, basic sciences, medicine, surgery, public health, libraries, obstetrics and gynecology, pediatrics, hospital administration, and radiology.

The fellowship program ramped up gradually and was in operation through 1973, by which time it was granting approximately fifty fellowships per year. The reason for ending the fellowship program was two-fold. Under new CMB president Dr. Patrick Ongley, the foundation set new goals in 1973, specifically with a sharper focus on empowering Asian institutions. At the same time, IRS tax rules in the United States changed, no longer allowing the "return home" provision. With concern over contributing to brain drain in regards to the overall objectives of the fellowships, Ongley modified the program and eventually moved the funds to block grants and matching grants.

Visiting Professorships

Visiting professorships were funded to foster mutual understanding between East and West, as well as the progress of medicine. Professors of a variety of specializations—medicine, pathology, orthopedic surgery, parasitology, physiology, public health nursing, bacteriology, and pharmacology—were sponsored to spend short (two- to six-month) or longer (two- or three-year) periods of time in

Table 1.2. CMB Fellowships 1951–1973 (Country Distribution).

Country	Travel Fellowships*	Study Fellowships	Total Fellowships
Japan	66	120	186
Taiwan	37	148	185
Thailand	12	94	106
South Korea	5	95	100
Philippines	13	54	67
Hong Kong	11	37	48
Indonesia	13	15	28
Singapore	7	19	26
Malaysia	4	19	23
Burma	4	2	6
USA	1	3	4
Fiji	0	3	3
Ceylon	0	1	1
Pacific Trust Territory	0	1	1
TOTAL	173	611	784

Source: CMB Annual Report 1972–1973, 22.
*The award of travel fellowships was discontinued in 1969.

residence in an Asian university's faculty of medicine. CMB sponsorship of visitors in the Far East started in 1952, with the first three visiting professors going to three medical schools in Taiwan, the Philippines, and Singapore. In 1957, the first year CMB annual reports began to list fellows and visitors by name and institutional affiliation, ten professors were visiting at faculties of medicine and schools of nursing throughout the region—including the Philippines, Japan, Taiwan, Thailand, Hong Kong, Burma, and Indonesia. As with the fellowship program, 1973 was the final year of the visiting professor program.

Medical Libraries

Importantly, CMB funded the rebuilding of medical school libraries that had been destroyed during the war years, assisting with restoration and reconstruction efforts. At the time, it prioritized the rehabilitation and strengthening of medical libraries, which extended not only to the purchasing of hundreds upon hundreds of books and journals, textbooks, and reference books for nursing and medical schools but also to the physical buildings that housed the library collections themselves. Remarkably, its funding made possible the opening of the only medical library in the Philippines in June 1953. CMB placed such importance on journal subscriptions that it enabled the gifting of institutional subscriptions to the Association of American Medical College's *Journal of Medical Education* to medical schools throughout the world, and it even continued its collection and storage of journal subscriptions meant for PUMC in hopes that someday it would be able to return and distribute them there. It also funded the translation of nursing textbooks into Chinese to fill a longstanding need, since almost no textbooks for nurses in Chinese were in existence in the early 1950s. The provision of medical books and journals was a key means by which CMB continued its promotion of medical education in the Far East.

Equipment and Supplies for Laboratories

During this period, CMB also gave grants more directly in aid of teaching and research, such as laboratory apparatus, surgical instruments, and teaching equipment for preclinical and surgical laboratories. These teaching and research grants included scientific equipment such as twenty microscopes for Siriraj Medical College in Bangkok and anesthesia apparatus that allowed for the establishment of the first training center in modern anesthesia in Japan.[3] CMB also facilitated the shipment of donated scientific equipment and teaching materials. Equipment and supplies for medical schools covered a wide range of scientific instruments for research—X-ray equipment, hematology laboratories, operating microscopes, tissue culture, and pathology and toxicology instruments, to name a few.

Other Funding Areas

CMB also gave funds for construction and building renovation due to damage sustained during World War II or the Korean War—for example, a grant to Yonsei University (formerly Severance Union Medical College) for a new medical sciences building. Grants were also made for teaching programs and research, including public health, nursing, preventative medicine, and basic science departments.

In sum, the first half of the 1950s saw CMB turning an exodus into an opportunity. In the early days of its new program, Dr. Harold Loucks, a former resident at PUMC and its Head of the Department of Surgery, became CMB director in 1954. By the spring of 1955, China Medical Board, Inc. changed its name to China Medical Board of New York, Inc. to eliminate any confusion or misunderstanding relating to its identity, as it continued to maintain its headquarters in New York City, and also committed itself to a primary aim of developing at least one medical college in each country into a satisfactory teacher-training center for that country.[4] Five years after its program in China abruptly came to a halt, CMB's projects ranged from the aforementioned four areas to other priority interest areas as diverse as midwifery training and tropical medicine. By this time, after CMB Director Harold Louck's first visit to Vietnam, it also found itself increasingly concerned with the problems of medical education in Southeast Asia.

In the mid-1950s, CMB supported two medical education conferences—the first Thai conference on medical education in 1956 and a conference on medical education for foreign scholars at the University of Wisconsin in 1957—to foster US-Asia exchange on medical education. Over one-third of the fifty foreign scholars who participated were Asian. Vietnam became a CMB grantee country in 1956. That same year, Dr. Oliver R. McCoy became assistant director, beginning his seventeen-year career with CMB. After Dr. Loucks' retirement in 1959, Dr. McCoy became CMB's director and president.

In the 1960s, under Dr. McCoy, CMB's program funding began to be redirected due to different paces of economic development—toward countries in which support was most needed and away from countries that had achieved self-sufficiency. For example, while funding decreased for Japan over time, funding increased to South Korea. In the 1960s, Taiwan was the most highly funded country in East Asia in terms of overall CMB grants—24 percent of total grant dollars—and in the 1970s, South Korea took its place with 28 percent (see Table 1.3). When CMB returned to China in the 1980s, grants to East Asia sharply declined when China overwhelmingly again became the funding priority, receiving 63 percent of its total grant funding over that decade.

In the 1960s, the second decade of CMB's program in East Asia, the top three areas of funding were institutional infrastructure development, faculty development, and capital projects and buildings. In a 1967 review of its Far East program, CMB decided to continue to support medical education and teacher training programs in medicine, nursing, and public health, focusing on increasingly fewer schools and instituting a requirement for grantees to match funds, up to 10 or 50 percent of the amount of the grant. In addition to those in the East Asian countries in Table 1.3, CMB continued to fund programs in the Philippines, Vietnam, Singapore, Indonesia, Thailand, Malaysia, and the United States. By the end of the decade, its portfolio included grants for supplies and equipment, teaching programs, library support, construction, and increased funding earmarked for individual research projects as a means to strengthen medical school faculties.

Table 1.3. East Asia Country Distribution of Grant Funding by Decades (Percent Distribution).

	1951–1960	1961–1970	1971–1980	1981–1990
China	7%	0%	0%	63%
Hong Kong	5%	4%	6%	3%
Japan	13%	14%	0%	0%
South Korea	8%	18%	28%	7%
Taiwan	13%	24%	12%	4%

Source: Norris 2003, 264–65 (Appendix I-4).

The beginning of the 1970s saw CMB continue its mission to improve the quality of medical, public health, and nursing education. By this time it was concentrating its support on one or more leading schools with the expectation that these schools would produce leaders to train others and elevate standard levels country-wide. In 1972, to continue to strengthen and encourage research projects, the first block grants for research were awarded to Siriraj Faculty of Medicine at Mahidol University, Seoul National University, and Yonsei University. Block grants gave greater flexibility and autonomy to the grantees in that they enabled researchers to select their own projects.

In 1973, Patrick Ongley succeeded Dr. McCoy as president. Soon after, CMB conducted a review of its program since 1951, followed by major program and funding changes. The first major program shift, due in part to the aforementioned newly introduced IRS regulations, phased out the twenty-year-old fellowship program. CMB became removed from the fellowship selection process, and so, for the first time, decisions and grant administration were shifted to its grantee institutions.

It was decided that CMB's future direction should focus on assisting local institutions in improving health services and on improving the quality and increasing the numbers of appropriate health care professionals. Its grant activities shifted to the following four areas: regional development in East and Southeast Asia, continuing education, delivery of health care, and development-fund grants. It stopped procuring materials and sending them to Asia, and instead gave larger grants to institutions to procure their own materials. The shift to regional development was to encourage the pooling of teaching and development resources within and between countries in Asia and to create space for grantees to analyze and approach their problems and implement their goals. CMB's Bill Sawyer later reflected on this period:

> We became partners, rather than parents. We were no longer paternalistic [toward grantees] and that transition was critical. Early in this 50-year period, the board still bought everything and shipped it. If they needed a box of microscope slides, they had a big staff that bought the slides and sent them to wherever. [When] we became partners . . . it changed the staff and the organization and the expenses of the board and turned it in to a cooperative thing where funds were made available. But our partner did the decisions and the purchasing and the management of those resources. And that is a massive transition for everybody. And I think that having worked in both systems, it's far better to be a partner. You can decide together but let them [grantees] be the owners, the operator, the decision makers after you have agreed to support them. It's very important. Pat Ongley really started that transition and had pretty well completed it by the time I came on board. . . . We tried to build on that and make it grow. (Norris 2003, 64)

As president, Ongley emphasized grants for institution building, changing CMB from an operating foundation and shifting its programs to medicine, nursing, public health education, research, and staff development. During this period, CMB also fostered the development of a network of national and regional training centers in Asia. It started providing support to schools for faculty training with the stipulation that these schools carry out training programs on a national basis. Starting in Thailand and Korea and extending, for example, to Singapore, support was given to national nursing education and training programs and regional fellowships.

In 1974, in line with its mission to advance local capacity, CMB instituted endowment grants (also known as development funds) to provide equal matching funds to schools to stimulate expansion of research capability. The first of these were given to the University of Hong Kong and to the College of Nursing at Yonsei University. Rather than giving direct research grants, as was done previously, matching grants made university faculties responsible for grant planning and evaluation. In order to raise money, grantee schools also engaged in fundraising and created alumni associations. CMB would give a sum to be matched from local resources, and the two would be combined as matching funds with restrictions. For the first five years, the principal was not available and only the income could be used to support research projects selected by the faculty's appointed committees. After another five years, the remaining half of the principal would become available. A CMB trustee at the time, explaining the decision to switch to this mode of making grants, commented:

> Our feeling was that the policy we had set was not the correct one. We should not try to make the [Asian grantee institutions] as much like us, but we should give them freedom to do what they wanted to do. Secondly, we should, as a Board, emphasize our support as working to help the people of [Asia] rather than build another ivory tower of medicine. And then our grants began to be first, more and more, 'What do you folks want to do?' in these various schools—and we'll help you with that—and second, what can be done to improve the health of the [Asia] people, particularly in medicine and in public health. (Norris 2003, 75)

And so, for over three decades outside mainland China, CMB funded a wide range of activities aiming at strengthening medical education throughout Asia. This broad spectrum included institutional infrastructure development, faculty development, capital projects, libraries, and biomedical research, as well as medical, nursing, and public health education. Trends in types of support shifted with leadership transitions within the foundation, as well with the changing political and socioeconomic conditions over time in the countries in which CMB was engaged. By the late 1970s, support in many Asian countries was no longer as critical as it had once been—including in South Korea and Hong Kong—and China was starting to open its door to the outside world. In 1979, with China's opening to the West, President Ongley visited China to set the groundwork for CMB's return.

Return to China: 1981—2014

In 1980, CMB accepted the government's invitation to return to China and broadened its work from a single medical college to partnerships with universities throughout the country. Two Chinese influential medical leaders (both also former presidents of PUMC), Huang Jiasi and Wu Jieping, were instrumental in the early days in supporting CMB's establishment of a relationship with the Chinese Ministry of Health. By 1981, CMB had initiated the funding of eight leading medical schools, including PUMC. CMB has since expanded its support of medical education and research to more than two dozen medical universities in China. It also remains active today in the Mekong countries of Southeast Asia, supporting medical universities to strengthen education and research in medicine, nursing, and public health in Cambodia, Laos, Myanmar, Thailand, and Vietnam.

During the early years of CMB's return to China, under the presidency of Patrick Ongley, matching grants and endowment funds were the primary forms of funding. With funds matched by the Chinese government, these grants created permanent endowments for the grantee institutions. The first set of such grants were endowment funds for staff development to establish six endowment funds of $500,000 each: $250,000 contributed by CMB and matched by the Chinese Ministry of Public Health. It was expressly stated in the grant appropriation that staff development was a major priority after China's thirty-year period of isolation from the West, development that was not merely to advance the careers of those trained but also to improve their institutions through better teaching and research.[5] This went hand in hand with CMB's fellowship funds for postgraduate education overseas. Again, as with the earlier Asian fellowships, the consequences of and many factors that contribute to "brain drain" were a concern.

After 1981, in its first decade in China, CMB gave the lion's share of its grants to the country—almost five times the rest of East Asia combined. While Japan's funding completely stopped in the early 1970s, Chinese institutions were granted over $25 million between 1981 and 1991, although funding for Korea, Taiwan, and Hong Kong dropped to $2.7 million, $1.5 million, and 1 million, respectively. During this period, China was receiving 63 percent of CMB's total funding and Thailand 16 percent, with the remaining 21 percent split among East Asian (7 percent to Korea, 4 percent to Taiwan, and 3 percent to Hong Kong) and Southeast Asian countries, including Indonesia, the Philippines, and Singapore (Norris 2003, 264). During this period, CMB started fostering regional exchanges with national and regional training centers in Asia such as interregional nursing programs in training centers in Hong Kong and Thailand.

While President Ongley shepherded in an era of new cooperation in China, helping schools to build their endowments, when Dr. Bill Sawyer became the next CMB president in 1988, he built on that legacy and moved in a new direction. Sawyer shifted from general funding to project funding based on the strengths and needs of each institution, focusing on advancing the level of scholarship and the quality of teaching and research facilities. Moreover, CMB began to see itself as an important source of "venture capital," meaning that it could fund promising, but more risky, projects that would have been difficult to attract matching funds from the government. During the Tiananmen Square events in 1989, it became concerned about the sustainability of its work amid the political instability, but in the end, CMB decided not to withdraw or curtail its activities in China, on the rationale that the role of medicine should be apolitical (Norris 2003, 143). Around the same time, Sawyer started convening the presidents of grantee universities, which provided an opportunity for school leaders to get together informally and talk about mutual concerns. CMB has continued this tradition with annual or biannual "President's Council" meetings as a forum for exchange of information between the CMB president and the presidents of grantee institutions.

Operating during the period of China's opening up, "CMB decided that it would not crusade for social change, but it would crusade for improving health by upgrading education and research" (Norris 2003, 123). The 1990s saw an even stronger pull of grant funds toward China, with the country receiving 87 percent of CMB's total grants over the decade. By this time, CMB had, for the most part, shifted out of East Asia and into Laos and Vietnam, also adding new grantee schools in Mongolia and Nepal and helping to establish Tibet Medical College from a provincial training school. In 1990, CMB was invited by the Myanmar government to visit the country, making it the first nongovernmental organization to be invited to the country in over thirty years. Over the decade, Myanmar became CMB's second most funded country after China, with $2.5 million (Norris 2003, 177).

In 1994, CMB started the Program of Higher Nursing Education Development (POHNED) to foster interregional cooperation and help elevate the profession of nursing with an exchange program for nursing training at universities in Xi'an and Chiang Mai. In addition to nursing, CMB funding areas in the 1990s in medical and public health education included curriculum reform, biomedical research, and clinical skills, with a growing emphasis on rural and minority populations and community medicine. It also had a marked increase in grants for telecommunications, since economic growth, the rise of the internet, and globalization were rapidly changing the environment in which CMB was doing its work.

After Roy Schwarz became CMB president in 1997, he led major programs in telemedicine to connect resource-poor schools to resources in teaching and research. In 1999, CMB established the Institute for International Medical Education (IIME) for defining the essentials of and developing standards for undergraduate medical programs. The Global Minimum Essential Requirements (GMER) included medical knowledge, clinical skills, and professional attitudes, behavior, and ethics.

Under the current president, Lincoln Chen (2007–present), CMB launched a fresh initiative to strengthen scientific excellence in critical capacities among Chinese and Asian institutions so as to promote equitable access to primary and preventive health services. This initiative refocused CMB's grants into three major program areas: building capacity in health professional education, advancing the field of health policy and systems sciences, and national capacity-building and regional health cooperation in Southeast Asia, including Cambodia, Laos, Myanmar, Thailand, and Vietnam. In 2010, President Chen launched a dialogue on health education reform in Asia with *The Lancet*'s Commission Report on Health Professionals for the Twenty-First Century, which has generated national medical education reform movements (Frenk et al. 2010). In 2011, CMB established a representative office in Beijing to more deeply engage with its Chinese partners. While English is the working language of CMB and its grantee institutions, communications have been strengthened with staff who are based in Asia and fully bilingual. In 2015, due to the realization that CMB's funding capacity has become relatively small in the context of China and Southeast Asia's growing wealth and in order to meet the challenges of a new era and to stretch limited budgets, it shifted to a direct operating foundation, allowing it to harness social and intellectual capital to augment is financial resources.

CMB's Second Century

CMB celebrated its centennial anniversary in 2014, giving thanks for one hundred years of partnerships, cooperation, and friendships since it was established by the Rockefeller Foundation in 1914. Initially founded to support just one medical school in China, in over a century of philanthropy, CMB has helped to catalyze health progress throughout Asia, provided $1.5 billion to over 100 medical universities, supporting thousands of individual fellows and funding innovations in research and education throughout a distinct three-phase history (1914–1950, 1951–1980, and 1981–2014).

As CMB embarks on its second century of harnessing knowledge for good health, it confronts a new set of challenges as the health, economic, and political contexts for CMB's work are rapidly changing. China and Asia, like much of the industrialized world, are experiencing the triple tsunamis of population aging, noncommunicable diseases (NCDs), and the growing burden of disability. In responding to these rapidly evolving challenges, all countries are struggling with health care access, quality, safety, and escalating costs, and these demographic and epidemiologic transitions will call for fundamentally different health and educational systems. How well are health professionals in China and Asia preparing for these shifts? How will decisions made in one country affect the health of its neighbors? How can much-needed reforms in delivery of health services and health professional education support each other? Can new technologies provide the tools and momentum that place learners at the center of education? As opportunities are opening to overcome some of these obstacles, CMB will continue support for regional networks and building capacity in educating health professionals. It will also continue support for policy research in priority areas such as postgraduate medical education for general-practitioner training, rural health, and nursing. As it moves into its second century of philanthropy, CMB is continuing its legacy of pioneering by strategic investments in emerging fields such as e-learning, global health, and health equity.

Annex. CMB Grantee Institutions 1951–2000*

Source: Norris 2003, Appendix J
*Between these years, CMB also gave grants to institutions in Cambodia, China, Ceylon, Indonesia, Laos, Malaysia, Mongolia, Myanmar, Nepal, the Philippines, Thailand, and Vietnam.

Hong Kong

University of Hong Kong

Japan

Chiba University Medical School
Gifu Prefectural Medical College
Gunma University Medical School
Hirosaki University Medical School
Hiroshima University Medical School
Hokkaido University Medical School
Hyogo Prefectural Medical School
Iwate Medical College
Juntendo Medical College
Kagoshima Prefectural Medical College
Kanazawa University Medical College
Keio University Medical School
Konee-Cho Yoshida
Kumamoto University Medical School
Kurume University Medical School
Kyoto Prefectural Medical College

Kyushu University Medical School
Mie Medical College
Nagasaki University Medical School
Nagoya City University Medical School
Nara Prefectural Medical College
Niigata University Medical School
Nippon Medical College
Okayama University Medical School
Osaka Medical College
Sapporo Medical College
Shinshu University Medical School
Showa Medical College
Toho Medical College
Tohoku University Medical School
Tokushima University Medical School
Tokyo Jikei Medical School
Tokyo Medical College
Tokyo Medical and Dental University
Tokyo University Medical School
Tokyo Women's Medical College
Tottori University Medical School
Wakayama Medical College
Yamaguchi University Medical School
Yokohama Municipal University

South Korea

Chonnam University Medical College
College of Medicine of Seoul National University
Ewha Medical College
Kyung-Puk University
Pusan National University
School of Public Health, Seoul National University
Sudo Medical College
Yonsei University Medical College

Taiwan

National Defense Medical Center
National Taiwan University
Taipei Medical College
Takau Medical College

Notes

1. China Medical Board Annual Report of 1950–1951, 4.
2. China Medical Board Annual Report of 1951–1952, 3–4.
3. China Medical Board Annual Report of 1951–1952, 5.

4. China Medical Board Annual Report of 1954–1955, 9.
5. China Medical Board of New York, Inc. Minutes (1981–1983), 6/11/81: 81013.

References

China Medical Commission of the Rockefeller Foundation. 1914. *Medicine in China*. New York: Rockefeller Foundation.

Frenk, Julio, Lincoln Chen, Zulfiqar A. Bhutta, Jordan Cohen, Nigel Crisp, Timothy Evans, Harvey Fineberg, et al. 2010. "Health Professionals for a New Century: Transforming Education to Strengthen Health Systems in an Interdependent World." *The Lancet* 376: 1923–58.

Norris, Laurie. 2003. *The China Medical Board: 50 Years of Programs, Partnerships, and Progress (1950–2000)*. New York: China Medical Board.

2 American Medical Education and US Engagement in East Asia, 1950–1970

Jesse B. Bump and Paul J. Cruickshank

Introduction

American influence on medical education around the world is closely associated with the scientific transformation promoted by the Flexner Report of 1910, but it was decades later, during the 1950s and 1960s, that the United States reached the pinnacle of its global power. Although military and economic prowess at the height of the Cold War underlay strong international influence in many areas, scant attention has been directed toward understanding either the history of medical education in this period or the government's postwar attempts to link overseas medical research initiatives with foreign policy objectives. The present chapter provides a perspective on American medical education, medical research, and related overseas activities during the period and serves as a counterpart to other chapters that adopt a domestic focus on the development of medical education from Chinese, Japanese, Korean, and Taiwanese perspectives.

Against a backdrop of Cold War politics, rising American influence, and the *pax Americana* of the mid-twentieth century, three important trends in US medical education arose. First, medical schools were reoriented around a growing focus on biomedicine and basic research, as opposed to an earlier focus on clinical training. Second, the US federal government became a large and influential actor by providing funding and direction for research, primarily via the National Institutes of Health (NIH), and for clinical care, via the Medicare and Medicaid entitlement programs. Third, medical schools sought to temper their emphasis on basic research and biomedicine by expanding educational content and medical manpower around the actual burden of disease by launching community health centers, and developing training for nurses, physician assistants, and auxiliary health service providers.

This chapter also investigates attempts to export American ideas about health, medicine, and medical research to other parts of the world by tracing the larger story of how the US government confronted the postwar world with new agencies and programs in an attempt to spread its influence, particularly in health and medical policies. Special attention is paid to NIH as the dominant domestic player in medical research and to its Pacific Office in Tokyo, which was launched in 1962 with authority over all NIH programs in East Asia. From these vantage points, we discuss how both domestic politics and foreign policy shaped overseas engagement in medical education and research. In these episodes, we also trace the tension between strategic political goals, which tended to be the interest of Congress, and the scientific goals of researchers, who were expected to implement Congress's policies.

The Flexner Report and US Medicine in the Twentieth Century

Although reforms were underway earlier, the Flexner Report of 1910 has come to symbolize the wholesale redirection of US medicine from an unorganized, unregulated craft to a unified profession based in science and research, housed at universities, and controlled by its own oversight bodies with authority grounded in law (Barr 2011).

The Carnegie Foundation for the Advancement of Teaching commissioned and published Flexner's *Medical Education in the United States and Canada*, and its recommendations were later embraced and supported by the Rockefeller Foundation (Flexner 1910). The report called for a new model of medical education centered on scientific research and practiced at university medical schools and affiliated hospitals. Johns Hopkins was singled out as a model for others to follow. In addition, Flexner proposed that the medical profession be more tightly regulated and that its educational requirements should be advanced. These measures were designed to reduce the number of physicians and medical schools and advance the quality of those remaining. Flexner also advocated protecting his proposed standards through state legislation on medical practice licenses.

The transformation of US medical education occurred almost exactly as recommended by Flexner, although it was underway long before the report was commissioned, and Flexner himself guided much of that transformation after taking a series of positions at Rockefeller philanthropies (Barr 2011; Ludmerer 2011). Medical education became a postbaccalaureate graduate pursuit, medical schools rebuilt their curriculums around the German research model brought to the United States by Johns Hopkins, and the supply of physicians shrank while their specialized research capacities grew. The pre–World War II period unfolded largely along Flexner's template, with most independent, for-profit schools closing and the surviving university medical schools striving to increase their standards and train more of the new, research-oriented physicians (Ludmerer 1999).

Post–World War II: Research and Educational Developments

While the implementation of Flexnerian reforms defined the story of US medical schools in the interwar period, the US government redefined the scope, content, and meaning of medical education after World War II. In the immediate postwar decades, US medical education was fundamentally reoriented into biomedical research by government funding. Medical schools transformed to unabashedly become the site for explorations into the biochemical mechanisms of disease.

The government's turn toward sponsoring research and its concordant influence on medical education developed from the unique mix of postwar social mores, institutional arrangements, and personal relationships among the Washington, DC elite. For the American public, and government officials more generally, the war demonstrated that basic research could be leveraged to further the ends of the state and that the government should engage in basic research. Though nuclear weapons revealed the destructive power of science, wartime developments such as DDT, penicillin, and new vaccines showed that research could improve and extend lives (Packard 1997). This realization created a faith in technology and helped to foster the public sentiment that the government should fund research in science, especially as it relates to medicine. In this logic, sustained investment could extend the positive wartime record and develop new technological breakthroughs. Additionally, while national health insurance was not politically feasible, medical research and hospital construction easily won bipartisan support in Congress. Politicians balked at socialized medicine, but they gladly backed the government's support of research. And after the Russian launch of Sputnik, the US government's financial and political support of research in the physical and medical sciences only continued to increase. Essentially, the promise of the discovery of new cures framed biomedicine as a peacetime weapon: it could combat disease, buy health, and possibly delay death.

Federal Funding for Research

The sustained growth in funding of biomedical research—from US $87 million in 1947 to more than $2 billion in 1968—was made possible by a long-standing collaboration of a small number of politicians, lobbyists, and scientists both inside and outside the US government. Government scientists such as James Shannon of NIH went to great lengths in public and before Congress to highlight the potential and promise of medical research for the well-being of Americans. Wealthy Washington socialites, including Mary Lasker and Frances Mahoney, devoted their personal fortunes to the reelection campaigns of countless members of Congress who supported legislation for the continued fight against disease (Drew 1967). On Capitol Hill, members of Congress such as Senator Lister Hill and Representative John E. Fogarty controlled key committees for many years that ensured smooth passage of medical research legislation.

Previously an unknown and largely marginalized institution, NIH became the central conduit for the growth and development of biomedical research. It had begun in 1887 as a small bacteriology lab within the US Public Health Service (PHS). In 1930, the laboratory, by that point based in the capital, was reorganized as a stand-alone institution and renamed the National Institute of Health and began to focus on basic science research into disease etiology. In subsequent decades, additional institutes were added to NIH: between 1947 and 1966, twelve new institutes and centers were added, and the overall NIH budget increased from $8 million to $1 billion (National Institutes of Health). Each institute was oriented around specific disease problems or organ systems, and a portion of the new funding allocation would go toward laboratory research on NIH's campus.

However, much of the funding was actually given to scores of US medical schools that became unequivocally committed to research. The decision to support research outside of government laboratories was made possible through the development of new, unique funding mechanisms for health research. During World War II, Surgeon General Thomas Parran secured authority for the PHS, and thus NIH, to award grants for deserving research outside of its own government institutes (Appel 2000). Unlike that of the Office of Naval Research, the wartime hub of scientific funding, NIH funding determinations did not rest with governmental program officers but with committees of academic scientists called "study sections." These peer committees often comprised leading research scientists based at universities who, given their position in the center of their field's respective research communities, could (in theory) easily identify who was doing the best research and which institutions could support new programming. An interest in leveraging universities for national goals prevailed over the lingering suspicion of the possibility of federal money shaping academic research priorities.

For medical schools, the two decades following World War II were defined by the ascendancy of the researcher: the clinicians and instructors who had been central to medical education were supplanted by researchers with newfound financial support and influence. Governmental funding for medical research was not a new concept, but at this time, the scale grew at an unprecedented rate and nearly every school in the United States was touched by the new federal largesse.

For the largest and leading medical schools, new federal support fundamentally transformed them from teaching institutions to research institutes. New money supported expansion of physical plant size, graduate training programs, operating budgets, research specialties, and support staff. Grants were awarded to scientists themselves, increasing their salaries and adding to their political power as faculty, and medical schools themselves were directly rewarded with support for overhead costs and other various matching grants. From 1951 to 1966, "salaried faculty at US medical schools increased from 3,500 to more than 17,000" and the overall proportion of junior and senior faculty focused on biomedical research also increased (Ludmerer 1999, 145). Large-scale, rapid growth created some controversy, but by 1970, US medical schools were de facto large-scale research institutions that included a wide variety of basic scientists across several disciplines and lines of research inquiry.

The significance of these institutional changes was also felt in the content of the medical curriculum and the choices medical students could make about how to understand and treat disease. A Flexnerian curricular model stressing understanding of basic sciences was supplemented with an even greater emphasis on biomedicine. Foundational courses in biochemistry were increasingly taught by PhD specialists, and students were encouraged to enroll in new specialties, including immunology, genetics, and molecular biology (Ludmerer 1999). While clinical experimentation became more sophisticated and some physicians focused on clinical solutions for the patient's immediate needs at the bedside, the major pedagogical emphasis was on understanding the most basic biochemical mechanisms of illness through work in the research laboratory. Students and clinicians spent an increasing percentage of their time doing research in facilities comparable to or better than university science departments. It was not uncommon for students and residents to do six-month rotations in different laboratories or to spend one to two years pursuing their own research projects within their subspecialty. Though still proportionally a small minority, an increasing number of medical students pursued an additional basic science PhD to supplement their medical degree. In an era characterized by the development of cortisone, the polio vaccine, and new pharmaceutical discoveries, there was a widely held confidence in American medicine that experimental medicine through research into the basic sciences would lead to a new understanding and innovative treatments against many diseases.

Beyond the Flexner Model: Reform of Pedagogy and Clinical Practice

By the mid-1960s, leaders at several medical schools across the United States began promoting a new model for medical education. Until these new ideas, there was little attempt at actual reform of the Flexnerian model that had been widely disseminated in the 1910s and 1920s because new research funding from the government had extensive influence on medical education. To some degree, however, it was a continuation of core interests in science-based education. The changes of the 1960s were both the next step of Flexnerian reform and a break from its traditions, but they have received little attention historically due to predominant interest in the earlier reforms just after the turn of the twentieth century.

While the cogency and clarity of Flexner's critique was still praised by postwar educators, they also found its standardized curriculum too rigid. The deans and faculty of schools like Case Western Reserve University (CWRU), Stanford, and the University of California, Los Angeles (UCLA) began pioneering a new model that emphasized a wide variety of electives to supplement a smaller program of core required science classes (Field 1970). The electives would cover new scientific fields, further study in core fields, introductions to new subspecialties, and nonbiomedical courses in behavioral science, health policy, sociology, and history.

The rise of the core and elective model was driven by three factors. First, there was general agreement among schools that the Flexnerian model had successfully achieved its earlier objectives (ibid.). The standardized premedical education of basic science courses had worked, and students in postwar decades were arriving at medical school better prepared. Faculty thought that the overall quality of students was better and that the basic science content taught in the first year of medical school in the Flexner model could be revised and made more demanding.

Second, there was a sense of the exceptional growth of new knowledge and specialization as a result of the expansion of biomedical research (ibid.). Physicians and students alike felt overwhelmed by the amount of information needed to practice medicine. The knowledge of what was important for understanding diseases and treating patients was constantly changing, and the rapid growth of new knowledge about the biochemical mechanisms of disease only accelerated this change. This called into question what content and training would best prepare students to become successful physicians in the future. New, specialized knowledge could not be easily classified into existing disciplines, and new approaches to a disease would be fragmented and introduced across several courses. The faculty of UCLA and Stanford pushed for the introduction of specialized electives that would allow students to systematically and coherently introduce new research topics. These schools, as well as CWRU, introduced the core and elective model as a mechanism to allow specialized courses, but also to continually introduce more electives in the future without needing to readjust the curriculum when a new specialty arose.

Third, several influential postwar medical educators, including George Packer Berry, dean of Harvard Medical School, vigorously pushed for the restructuring of medical education to enable elective courses in social sciences, behavioral science, and the humanities. Such content would create a "comprehensive medicine" that would ensure that student physicians were well-rounded and able to appreciate social, political, and historical factors that influence disease and underlie the human condition (Berry 1953, 21). These concerns were not new; explicit interest in understanding the social determinants of disease alongside (or in place of) the biochemical mechanisms of disease has been present since the mid-nineteenth century. While the debate over adding these topics was extensive, this content was generally not included as electives in the 1950s and early 1960s (Field 1970).

The model of core science courses supplemented with electives was gradually adopted, school-by-school, without the influence of a nationwide report or foundational support to push for change. Educators, deans, and historians alike emphasized that this reform, like most all educational reform, was extremely difficult institutionally and could be accomplished only on a school-by-school basis and only through the use of significant political capital and support in the medical school, affiliated hospitals, and the university itself.

Clinical Teaching, Clinical Practice, and the Question of Medical Manpower

The new importance of benchtop research in the postwar period did not diminish the continued significance of clinical education. In fact, the two were more complementary than antagonistic. The wartime success of medical research and the fruits of postwar basic science helped to change Americans' perspective toward medical care. The American public came to hold physicians in increasingly high regard, and there was an overall rise in the demand for clinical care. For example, in 1934, the New York Hospital had 13,467 admissions and 189,571 days of patient care; in 1964, those numbers had risen to 28,459 admissions and 293,227 days of clinical care. Accounting for population growth over the same period suggests that the ratio of visits per person might have roughly doubled (Ludmerer 1999). Under these new circumstances, teaching hospitals had the highest reputation among both patients and practicing physicians: these wards had access to the best knowledge, the latest ideas, and students and residents trained in the newest practices.

While biomedicine was the focus of classroom and laboratory instruction, clinical instruction continued in its longstanding traditions of leveraging the "charitable" poor for student learning (Humphreys 2002, 514). Teaching hospitals in urban settings continued to use local neighborhoods for instruction, but low-income patients began to place an increasing financial burden on such hospitals as more technology was used in routine cases. This fiscal pressure coincided with teaching hospitals moving toward semiprivate care provision (i.e., shared treatment rooms) that could generate more revenue through the increasingly popular health insurance policies that developed in the 1950s. As a new constituency for students to learn from, these semiprivate patients had both advantages and disadvantages. On the one hand, middle and upper-middle class patients had a different burden of disease than the charitable poor, but on the other hand, they often refused treatment from students or new residents in favor of the seasoned attending physician (Irby, Cooke, and O'Brien 2010).

Whatever gradual shift there was toward semiprivate patients in the 1950s and 1960s was promptly reversed with the introduction of Medicare and Medicaid in the mid-1960s. Low-income patients that had once been a financial drain were now supported financially, and clinical practice became a "megabusiness" for clinical instructors. "Medical faculties expanded dramatically, and the primary income for medical schools became clinical practice revenue generated by the faculty" (ibid., 223). The institutional separation of teaching hospitals and medical schools, combined with the ability for dually appointed clinicians to draw a share of their salary from treating private patients, created a conflict. While new financial sources were celebrated in schools, some educators saw it as a threat: clinical instructors no longer had any time for teaching, and teaching hospitals and medical schools were continually at odds over the immediate care of patients versus the long-term instruction of students.

Another major impact on clinical education came from the changing burden of disease in the late 1960s and new perceptions about investments in health infrastructure. With the rising prevalence of chronic and behavioral diseases, educators, officials, students, and public commentators alike expressed grave concern over the realities of medical care for the general public: despite the protection of Medicaid/Medicare, the poor and elderly still had difficulty accessing care; services for the average patient were fragmented across a growing number of subspecialties; and growing investments in research focused on obscure diseases rather than prevention or public health. In response, medical students pushed for greater focus on community medicine, epidemiology, and general services that could meet typical, day-to-day patient needs. In part to help address these care delivery needs with more personnel, policymakers pushed to develop more training programs for nurses and physician assistants (Krevans and Condliffe 1970).

This last debate about the composition of the medical profession—specifically regarding the total number of physicians needed in the United States—was one of the more longstanding debates of twentieth-century medicine that connects directly back to Flexner. Implicit in the closure of unregulated medical schools was an argument that America had an "oversupply of poorly trained physicians" (Blumenthal 2004, 1781). With Flexnerian reforms for producing "fewer, but better doctors," the ratio of physicians to the general population fell from 173 per 100,000 in 1900 to 125 per 100,000 in 1930 (Starr 1984, 126). Commentators in subsequent years, especially economists, elaborated on various assumptions to argue for an over- or under supply of "medical manpower" and, thus, rationally regulate the total number of US medical students and physicians. In the midst of growing demand for care and an more affluent public, the most dire prognosis came from the 1959 Surgeon General's Consultant Group on Medical Education (the Bane Report), which predicted a shortage of over "40,000 physicians in the United States by 1975" (Blumenthal 2004, 1782). The Kennedy and Johnson administrations responded with legislation to subsidize medical schools, and from 1965 to 1980, the total number of US medical schools increased from 88 to 126, with the number of graduates expanding from 7,409 to 15,135 (Starr 1984, 421).

American Engagements with East Asia

Beginning early in the twentieth century, the Rockefeller Foundation (RF) played a pioneering role in spreading American ideas of health, medicine, and disease control to less developed parts of the world. For the most part, these activities were conducted through its International Health Division (IHD), which operated under slightly different names from 1913 until it was closed in 1951, and the China Medical Board (CMB), which was launched in 1914 and then spun off as a separate entity in 1928 (Farley 2004). Through these channels, the RF pursued its goals using two primary strategies. One was to build institutions, of which the Peking Union Medical College (PUMC) is a leading example (Bullock 1980). An important component of RF's institution-building was to build capacity through fellowship exchange programs. The other strategy was to focus on individual diseases, which sometimes coincided with wider institution-building efforts. Targeted diseases included hookworm, malaria, and yellow fever. Against yellow fever, RF's successes included eliminating the vector mosquito from northern Brazil, producing the first vaccine, and even coordinating production and administration of the vaccine to hundreds of thousands of British and American soldiers in World War II (Ettling 1981; Packard and Gadehla 1997; Rockefeller Foundation 2013b). But after the war, RF began to wind down its IHD, effectively closing it in 1951.

The fall of IHD corresponded roughly to the rise of the United States as an international superpower. The US government embraced this role with a raft of global initiatives. Cornerstones of the new American era were laid during and after World War II, including institutions to manage international trade, stabilize the world economy, rebuild Europe, and limit future military conflict—the General Agreement on Tariffs and Trade (now the World Trade Organization), the International Monetary Fund, the World Bank, and the United Nations, respectively. Through its leadership in designing these institutions and complementary bilateral initiatives such as the Marshall Plan, the United States spread its influence on an unprecedented scale.

In many ways, the end of RF's IHD reflected the dominance of its ideas and their absorption into mainstream US government programs and those of new multilateral institutions. What had been the focus of IHD became the province of the World Health Organization (WHO), which was founded in 1948 with a very similar mission. Furthermore, many former IHD staff took senior positions at WHO. As a direct consequence, WHO's first major program was in malaria eradication, an RF priority since 1915 (Packard 1998).

The expansion of US military, economic, and political influence soon translated to a more internationalist approach in many other areas, including in health and medicine. Agencies, laws, and programs to support international activities by the US government followed closely on the heels of the Bretton Woods institutions, the UN agencies, and the Marshall Plan. This included the Mutual Security Administration, in 1951, which, among many other things, funded malaria control projects for military and political reasons in Greece and Turkey.[1] The International Health Research Act of 1960—initially introduced as the Health for Peace bill (1958)—further supported these efforts for the purposes of promoting American health via research elsewhere and supporting international health science research (Congressional Record 1958; National Institutes of Health 2015).[2] The following year (1961), the Kennedy administration launched the US Agency for International Development as a permanent home for activities previously spread across many agencies, including the Mutual Security Agency, the Technical Cooperation Agency, the Foreign Operations Administration, and the International Cooperation Administration.[3]

The government increasingly recognized that development assistance activities were a crucial part of US foreign policy in the Cold War. While diverse institutions pushed a global vision of mutual support in international health, many organizations used medicine as a means of advancing political agendas. After the Soviet Union took the lead in the space race by launching the satellite *Sputnik* in 1957, US policymakers and business lobbies promoted their interests by referring to races of other kinds, all of which warranted US investment lest the Soviets notch more victories.

The perceived competition extended to health and medicine, where some feared that the Soviets would dispatch medicine, doctors, and other caregivers internationally to win hearts and minds. The Health for Peace bill and other US medical research initiatives of the time gained much of their impetus from their potential to advance the US position in the contest. If the Soviet Union had greater manpower, then perhaps the United States could compete with more specialized knowledge and more medicines. The official legislation broadening NIH's foreign activities had this motivation at its source (Tobbell 2009). As a comprehensive review of all federal support for research overseas observed in 1961, "research support programs can affect the conduct of foreign policy and the pursuit of political objectives abroad by engendering good or bad feelings toward the US and advancing or hindering the achievement of overall foreign policy objectives."[4]

Generally, the objectives of US support for research overseas fell into four categories, according to the review. First, foreign policy purposes included "influencing the attitudes and actions of other nations and peoples toward the US, or advancing the prestige, economic and political status, and influence of the US." Second, security objectives included research for military purposes. Third were the programmatic objectives of technical agencies. And fourth was the advancement of science for its own sake, "arising from the unity and universality of scientific endeavor."[5]

The growing awareness of research as a foreign policy instrument fostered tremendous expansion in NIH's international portfolio. In 1947, its international activities included just nineteen projects, involving a modest $179,000. Ten years later, in 1957, it had 224 international projects, backed by $1.8 million. By 1967, it had over 1,200 international projects and was spending more than $20 million per year to support them.[6] To provide some perspective on these sums, RF had spent a total of about $94 million on its international projects between 1913 and 1951 (Rockefeller Foundation 2013a). Adjusting for inflation based on the middle year (1932), versus 1965, suggests that, through the decade of the 1960s, NIH was spending, on average, about ten times more per year than had RF.

NIH also embraced RF's model of fellowships. Before the late 1950s, NIH funded visits to the United States by foreign postdoctoral fellows on the order of two or three dozen annually in most years, although there were none at all in 1955–1957. In the 1960s, there were between 150 and 180 such fellows every year, reflecting extra funding for this purpose available under the International Health Research Act (National Institutes of Health 2015). NIH also funded US medical scientists to visit foreign institutions. These fellowships also began modestly, with just one in 1947. But by 1957, there were eighty-six, and in the 1960s, there were two hundred to three hundred in most years, with nearly four hundred in 1966.[7]

These fellowships were important to fulfilling NIH's self-imposed "obligation" to "exercise leadership and join together with all nations on an international basis toward the advancement of the medical, biological, and behavioral sciences and in furthering the solution of disease, health, and social problems through research."[8] In part, the fellowships were intended to promote "more effective interchange of scientific workers throughout the world," which it was hoped would stimulate research and foster peace.[9]

In general, all fellows were expected to engage in normal scientific activities, including research, studying, learning, training, and mentoring. "After a year or two of training and experience in the US, the foreign scientists would return . . . with laboratory and clinical experience not available in their homelands and with first-hand knowledge of the scientific and other aspects of the culture of this country." Fellowships for Americans would "permit young scientists to go abroad for one or two years of study. . . . The advantages to be gained lie in the research opportunities and superior instruction . . . in certain specialized fields."[10]

In particular, many fellowships were arranged around specific US interests or problems of strategic importance. For instance, beginning in 1959, NIH administered a cholera research program in collaboration with the Southeast Asia Treaty Organization (SEATO). Operating with SEATO funding, the cholera research program began in Thailand and was later relocated to permanent headquarters in East Pakistan.[11] The program conducted epidemiological surveys of cholera, developed oral rehydration therapy (one of the twentieth century's most important medical innovations), and ultimately became the International Center for Diarrheal Disease Research, Bangladesh (ICDDR, B) (Ruxin 1994). Early projects were pursued in other countries of strategic Cold War interest as well, including Egypt, India, Indonesia, Israel, Poland, and Yugoslavia.[12]

Moves to expand NIH's international work were driven by strategic priorities that were not completely aligned. In keeping with its scientific and domestic roots, the initial expansion of international funding for the NIH was explicitly defined by domestic priorities. As its Director James Shannon of the NIH noted in a 1962 review of foreign activities:

> Since the primary objective of the NIH international program is to advance the status of the health sciences in the US, our grants are most frequently made in countries where adequate research resources are available and where original and productive ideas arise. This means that NIH relationships have been most extensive with the countries which are more advanced in the medical sciences, such as Canada, Japan, Australia, Israel, and the Western European countries. The fact that we do not frequently support scientists in newly-emerging countries also recognizes that their limited scientific manpower must not be diverted from the high-priority problems of that country by our support of projects of interest to us.[13]

NIH's scientific staff had been hired to pursue diseases of domestic importance, and they were unenthusiastic about international medical research and educational fellowships, which were pursued by Congress in the late 1950s and early 1960s for its own reasons.

Congressional interest in the late 1950s was spurred by President Eisenhower's calculated Cold War intelligence gathering through East-West scientific partnerships and "Works for Peace" campaigns. While early postwar international funding was directed at addressing domestic issues, legislation from the Kennedy administration onward was explicit in "winning the hearts and minds" of allies and nonaligned countries.[14] As the NIH formalized its international activities, it launched an Office of International Research in Bethesda, Maryland, alongside several international offices, including a Pacific Office based in Tokyo. These offices were an explicit part of US foreign policy and were intended to foster scientific progress, create goodwill, promote peace and security, and spread US influence during the Cold War. However, our analysis of NIH's Pacific Office records suggests that the general strategy was not translated into any specific actions. We did not find any evidence that the United States sought to build any institutions or focused on any countries for political reasons. Rather than building institutions, as did RF, NIH preferred instead to focus its overseas activities mainly on individual investigators, with notable exceptions such as WHO, which received some financial support.

NIH's Pacific Office in Tokyo was announced in late 1962 and began functioning soon thereafter, along with a satellite office in New Delhi. With oversight for East Asia, South Asia, and the Pacific, the Tokyo office's responsibilities included: representing NIH and advising grantees; collecting information on local capacities, problems, and needs; and making site visits to help assess proposals.[15]

Although Cold War considerations were clearly behind the international expansion of US research support, channeling political influence through the scientifically oriented NIH staff proved difficult. In Japan and other countries in the region, "it is predictable that these 'aid' aspects of NIH funding obscure its own fundamental objective in pursuing research," according to Pacific Office Chief Heinz Specht in 1964.[16] "If to this tendency we add the strong motivation of the Department of State to capitalize on any American participation in [foreign research], it is small wonder that NIH finds itself under very real pressure to 'guide' its conduct of research support by what are scientifically speaking irrelevant criteria," he complained. The result of bureaucratic impositions by both Bethesda and Washington was unclear policies, which the Tokyo office had difficulty explaining: "Of what possible use can it be to present these lame excuses to the scientific elite of other countries," Specht bridled in nine pages of withering criticism for attempts to privilege US interests—including US researchers—over matters of scientific merit.[17]

The international work of NIH, as seen in its global offices and broad disbursements for biomedical research, was further developed in the late 1960s with the creation of the Fogarty International Center (FIC). Styled as a research institute to coordinate transnational research funding, contextualize the global impact of biomedical science, and provide training for medical students and senior scientists alike, FIC became a way to highlight the positive international impact of US aid in light of negative sentiment toward US involvement in Vietnam.

It also became a space where government scientists and medical educators could focus on how training in biomedical research affected medical education globally. Training in experimental research fostered an important set of skills uniquely oriented to respond to the challenges of the 1960s and 1970s. This was an argument that cultivating scientific problem-solving abilities honed in biomedical research was the best long-term response for addressing the emerging and unpredictable transnational risks from pollution and social determinants of disease. By their logic, training in a lab was not an activity that would keep one away from the pressing needs of patients in developing countries. On the contrary, it would provide international health practitioners with the worldview, analytical rigor, and problem-solving skills to develop appropriate solutions for new problems as they arose (Condliffe and Furnia 1971, 18), regardless of geographical context. Experience in laboratory research, one of the key institutional and educational drivers in US postwar medical education, would foster an intellectual adaptability useful in any geographic context.

The shift in priorities in international funding for medical education and research—from the sponsorship of individual researchers to advanced training—largely mirrored US domestic concerns. The early postwar focus on supporting research reflected a similar domestic interest in understanding a shifting disease burden and leveraging the promise of medical science. Later, interests in the social determinants of disease, increased focus on biomedical science, and shifts in transnational medical education and care mirrored similar trends in the United States. By the early 1970s, the underlying policy concerns for medical education were about the same in scope, content, and relevancy as those of biomedically based medicine, in light of behavioral and chronic diseases increasingly affecting a stratified society.[18] Likewise, the relationship between technologically focused training via large institutions, on the one hand, and the actual needs of the population, on the other, was increasingly central to debates about medicine from the 1970s onward (Bryant 1969).

Although Specht's scathing memo from the Pacific Office shows the tensions between NIH's scientific mission and the political and administrative demands emanating from Washington, our review of records from the Pacific Office held by the National Archives found little evidence that overtly political activities were ever actually conducted through this channel. Monthly reports back to headquarters consisted almost entirely of summaries of Asian newspaper clippings concerning disease outbreaks, scientific and technical happenings, policies relating to health medicine or research, and associated administrative matters, including the founding of new universities and funding agencies. Reports of student unrest were common as well, but these were discussed in connection with their impact on supported projects, rather than with any greater political dimensions.[19]

At the macro level, the United States carefully and systematically planned the institutional architecture of the postwar world, but on the smaller scale of health and medical initiatives, we find a much more haphazard approach. Beyond rhetoric, the implementation of these initiatives does not seem to have been aligned well with US foreign policy goals, even as larger political and economic considerations constrained the underlying research mission in different ways. As a matter of administrative policy, America did not know how to prevent its research dollars from simply displacing spending by other governments.[20] And foreign governments had mixed reactions to US support, fearing it would create dependency on external resources.[21]

The expansion of foreign research support was driven by resources from an expanding US economy in the 1940s and 1950s, but by the late 1960s and early 1970s, balance-of-payment problems linked to the partial gold standard of the Bretton Woods agreements sharply curtailed the portfolio (Elwell 2011). (A balance-of-payments chart is available in appendix 2.) The consequences of these balance-of-payment problems were severe. "There is a continuing serious US balance of payments deficit problem. It is essential, therefore, that dollar expenditures overseas meet stringent criteria and be fully justified," wrote one administrator in 1972.[22] Particularly hard hit were research grants made overseas, since these exacerbated the balance-of-payments problem more than funding fellowships in the United States or expenses covered in local currencies generated through agricultural sales. In 1965, there were 801 foreign grants made by NIH, totaling about $11.5 million. By 1970, there were only 170, totaling just under $3 million.[23]

Conclusion

The larger history of the United States in the postwar period reveals the dominating influence of the Cold War contest for global hegemony on American policies at home and abroad. In waging this war, Americans continued the strategies that had underwritten victory in World War II. Many in governmental and academic circles believed that scientific research had turned the tide in the Allies' favor, particularly with radar and the atomic bombs, but also with myriad other innovations, including DDT for controlling insect-borne diseases and the mass production of penicillin. In the Cold War, the US government invested heavily in research and brought about the shift toward biomedicine.

In the domestic sphere, the federal commitment to research transformed medical education and medical research. First, in the search for wartime innovations and later, in response to federal funding, medical schools deemphasized clinical training in favor of biomedicine and basic research. The growth of this funding in the 1950s and 1960s, primarily through the National Institutes of Health, altered the balance of power in medical schools, favoring individual researchers over deans and other administrators. As the cost of clinical care provision rose, the government's response came in the form of Medicare and Medicaid entitlement programs, which created vast financial incentives for medical schools to provide care to the elderly and the poor. This renewed importance of clinical care in medical schools dovetailed with racial and social problems of the late 1960s. Both factors helped to reassert older concerns that had been overshadowed by the rise of biomedicine and basic research. Medical educators and researchers responded to these events by adding greater focus on patient-centered—as opposed to technology-centered—care and reemphasizing the role of the community and broad socioeconomic conditions in health and well-being. This shift also reflected the growing importance of behavior-related diseases, such as those caused by tobacco smoking, and the challenges of translating general scientific findings into local health outcomes. These changes in patients and disease burdens revived another older discussion concerning the appropriate mix of medical manpower and led to more training programs for nurses, physician assistants, and auxiliary health service providers.

Throughout the 1950s and 1960s, Cold War politics also strongly influenced US foreign policy. The US interventionist stance extended beyond core elements such as military and trade initiatives to include medicine and research as instruments of soft power (Nye 1990). The attempt to link domestic research prowess with foreign policy goals stemmed from a version of the arms race in which medical research was envisioned as a means to contest Soviet influence. Testifying to the depth of this effort were thousands of grants, totaling over $100 million in the 1960s alone, and the establishment of research support offices around the world, including the Pacific Office in Tokyo.

The rising economic and political power of the United States cut both ways. On the one hand, American expertise, resources, and leadership implied correctly that the United States had knowledge and money to share and a perspective from which other nations could learn. But on the other hand, the emergence of the American world order was so swift that many questions remained as to exactly what America sought to achieve and how it would do so. In health and medicine, it was obvious that US congressional priorities often reflected narrow US interests informed by politics and economics rather than the humanitarian language in which they were cloaked. Diseases on which America focused were those of military importance, such as cholera and malaria. For instance, when America made malaria a central focus of its international strategy in the late 1940s, 1950s, and 1960s, it did so primarily on the basis of economics. However, the larger geopolitical strategy that yielded funds for medical education and research was not necessarily embraced by the educators and scientists who were expected to actually implement specific programs. In our review of activities at NIH's Pacific Office in Tokyo, we found that US research staff contested priorities from Washington, hoping to assert instead the primacy of scientific merit. This example shows some of the complex factors and mixed motives that surrounded the attempted diffusion of ideas.

This US perspective on medical education and life science research highlights the importance of historical perspectives for explaining and contextualizing broad developments. This lens of US domestic processes and their influence on the government's engagement with East Asia reveals the broad questions that each local government had to confront in ways that were sometimes similar to and sometimes different from the US approach: what the appropriate balance of research, teaching, and patient care was and how authority derived from biomedical research could confront social issues and their influence on health. Furthermore, if this chapter highlights the American view, it is only one part of the larger picture of how these actions and ideas were received in East Asia, where they were (in various measures) rejected, modified, accepted, or interpreted within vastly different traditions and institutions of health and medicine.

Appendix 1: National Archives File Indexes

NARA 1: Record Group 443, UD-06D/Entry 1—Subject Files, Box 55, Folder O+M 2-V FIC Organization 1959–1972.
NARA 2: Record Group 443, UD-06D/Entry 1—Subject Files, Box 55, Folder O+M 2-V FIC Organization 1973–1982.
NARA 3: Record Group 443, UD-06D/Entry 1—Subject Files, Box 141, Folder INTL 1 International Organizations Dealing with Medical Research 1942–1971.
NARA 4: Record Group 443, UD-06D/Entry 1—Subject Files, Box 142, Folder INTL 2-1-B NIH Pacific Office (Tokyo) 1946–1976.
NARA 5: Record Group 443, UD-06D/Entry 1—Subject Files, Box 143, Folder INTL 3 International Health Activities Supported by NIH 1959–1971.
NARA 6: Record Group 443, UD-06D/Entry 1—Subject Files, Box 143, Folder INTL 3 International Health Activities Supported by NIH 1972–1977.

Appendix 2: US Balance of Payments by Year

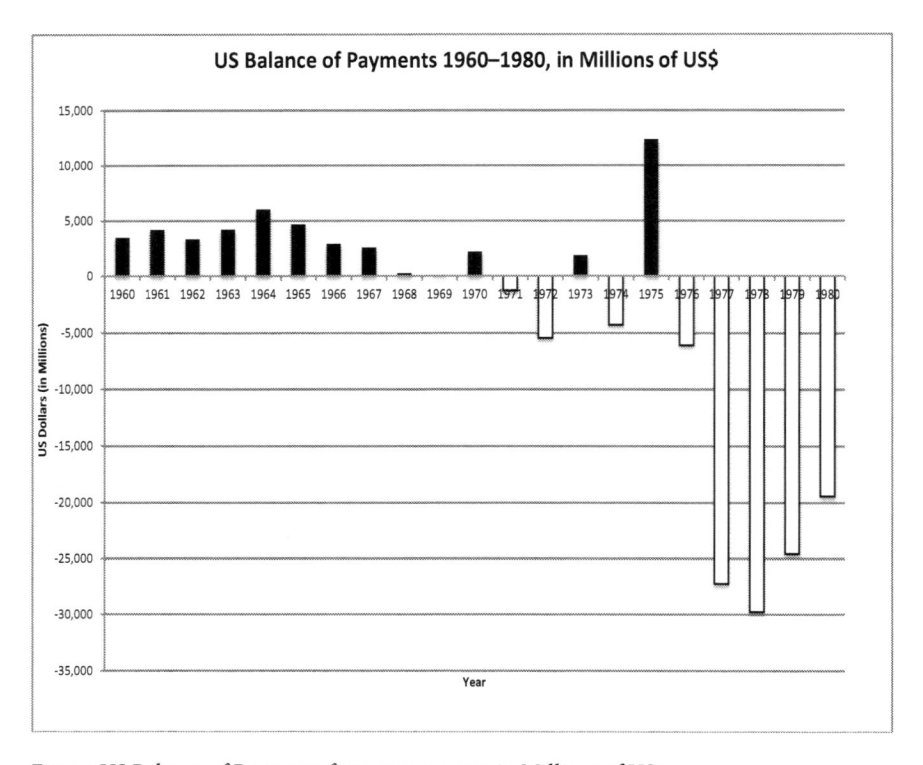

Fig. 2.1 US Balance of Payments from 1960 to 1980 in Millions of US$.
Source: Data from US Census Bureau, Economic Indicator Division 2015.

Notes

1. The records are available at the National Archives, http://www.archives.gov/research/guide-fed-records/groups/469.html.
2. See also "Summary of NIH International Activities," in NARA 5.
3. http://www.archives.gov/research/guide-fed-records/groups/469.html.
4. "The Support of Research in Foreign Countries by Agencies of the Federal Government," April 12, 1961, p. 9, in NARA 3.
5. Ibid., pp. 3–4.
6. All figures are from the Statistical Reference Book of International Activities, Fiscal Year 1972 Funds, DHEW Publication No. (NIH) 73-64, in NARA 6.
7. Ibid.
8. Part II: The Objectives and Functional Programs of the International Center, document NIH-OD-OPP 10/9/67, p. 3, in NARA 1.
9. Director, NIH to Surgeon General, March 28, 1958, "Medical Research—an International Program" in NARA 3.
10. Director, NIH to Surgeon General 28 March 28, 1958, "A Proposal for an Expanded International Program in the Life Sciences," section II, p. 6, in NARA 3.
11. International Activities of the National Institutes of Health, Fiscal Year 1961, March 17, 1961, in NARA 5.
12. Ibid.
13. James A. Shannon, "Special Report: The Impact of NIH International Activities Abroad," January 31, 1962, p. 3, in NARA, box 142, folder 1 "INTL 2-1 NIH Office of International Research 1960–1968."
14. See, for example, Senator Lister Hill (AL), "Health for Peace," Congressional Record 104 (January 23, 1958), S777.
15. Press Release HEW-V35, Thursday, October 4, 1962, in NARA 4.
16. "A View of NIH Policy from the NIH-Tokyo Office," September 30, 1964, p. 2, in NARA 4.
17. Ibid, p. 3.
18. It is worth noting that the debates about medical education in East Asia and, more generally, the international development of medical training were largely absent from the most prominent medical journals of the postwar decades. Keyword searches for "China," "Japan," "Taiwan," "South Korea," and "Hong Kong" in the *Journal of the American Medical Association* and the *Journal of Medical Education* returned articles focused on disease outbreaks in these areas or biographic profiles of US physicians practicing overseas. In a sense, the lack of visibility of this issue highlights that there was never a coherent overarching policy or strategy connecting the mainstream US profession with the interests and policies of the US Government and the various philanthropies and institutions interested in domestic and international medical education.
19. Some monthly reports available in NARA 4 (there is no complete collection).
20. "The Support of Research in Foreign Countries by Agencies of the Federal Government," April 12, 1961, p. 7, in NARA 3.
21. Memo from Associate Director for Extramural Research and Training of NIH to Files, March 10, 1972, in NARA 6.
22. Memo from Assistant Secretary for Health and Scientific Affairs RE Obligation Ceilings for International Transactions in FY 1972 and FY 1973, April 6, 1972, in NARA 6.
23. Statistical Reference Book of International Activities, Fiscal Year 1972 Funds, DHEW Publication No. (NIH) 73–64, in NARA 6.

References

Appel, Toby A. 2000. *Shaping Biology: The National Science Foundation and American Biological Research, 1945-1975*. Baltimore, MD: Johns Hopkins University Press.

Barr, D. A. 2011. "Revolution or Evolution? Putting the Flexner Report in Context." *Medical Education* 45 (1): 17-22.

Berry, G. P. 1953. "Medical Education in Transition." *Journal of Medical Education* 28 (3): 17-42.

Blumenthal, David. 2004. "New Steam from an Old Cauldron—The Physician-Supply Debate." *New England Journal of Medicine* 350 (17): 1780-87.

Bryant, John. 1969. *Health and the Developing World*. Ithaca, NY: Cornell University Press.

Bullock, Mary Brown. 1980. *An American Transplant: The Rockefeller Foundation and Peking Union Medical College*. Berkeley: University of California Press.

Condliffe, Peter G., and Arthur H. Furnia, eds. 1971. *Reform of Medical Education: The Role of Research in Medical Education*. Bethesda, MD: National Institutes of Health.

Drew, Elizabeth B. 1967. "The Health Syndicate: Washington's Noble Conspirators." *Atlantic Monthly* 220: 75-82.

Elwell, Craig K. 2011. "Brief History of the Gold Standard in the United States." Congressional Research Service 41887.

Ettling, J. 1981. *The Germ of Laziness: Rockefeller Philanthropy and Public Health in the New South*. Cambridge, MA: Harvard University Press.

Farley, John. 2004. *To Cast Out Disease: A History of the International Health Division of the Rockefeller Foundation (1913-1951)*. New York: Oxford University Press.

Field, John. 1970. "Medical Education in the United States: Late Nineteenth and Twentieth Centuries." In *The History of Medical Education: An International Symposium Held February 5-9, 1968*, ed. Charles Donald O'Malley, 501-30. Berkeley: University of California Press.

Flexner, Abraham. 1910. "Medical Education in the United States and Canada Bulletin Number Four" (The Flexner Report). New York: The Carnegie Foundation for the Advancement of Teaching.

Hill, Senator Lister (AL). 1958. "Health for Peace," Congressional Record 104 (January 23), S777-78.

Humphreys, Margaret. 2002. "Time to Heal: American Medical Education from the Turn of the Century to the Era of Managed Care (Review)." *Journal of the History of Medicine and Allied Sciences* 57 (4): 514-15.

Irby, David M., Molly Cooke, and Bridget C. O'Brien. 2010. "Calls for Reform of Medical Education by the Carnegie Foundation for the Advancement of Teaching: 1910 and 2010." *Academic Medicine* 85 (2): 220-27.

Krevans, Julius R., and Peter G. Condliffe. 1970. *Reform of Medical Education: The Effect of Student Unrest*. Washington, DC: National Academy of Sciences.

Ludmerer, K. M. 1999. *Time to Heal: American Medical Education from the Turn of the Century to the Era of Managed Care*. New York: Oxford University Press.

———. 2011. "Abraham Flexner and Medical Education." *Perspectives in Biology and Medicine* 54 (1): 8-16.

National Institutes of Health. "World War II Research and the Grants Program." National Institutes of Health. Accessed August 10, 2016. https://history.nih.gov/exhibits/history/docs/page_06.html.

———. 2015. "Legislative Chronology: 1960." National Institutes of Health. Accessed August 10, 2016. https://history.nih.gov/research/sources_legislative_chronology.html#1960.

Nye, Joseph S. 1990. *Bound to Lead: The Changing Nature of American Power.* New York: Basic Books.
Packard, Randall M. 1997. "Visions of Postwar Health and Development and Their Impact on Public Health Interventions in the Developing World." In *International Development and the Social Sciences*, edited by Frederick Cooper and Randall Packard, 93–115. Berkeley: University of California Press.
———. 1998. "'No Other Logical Choice': Global Malaria Eradication and the Politics of International Health in the Post-War Era." *Parassitologia* 40 (1–2): 217–29.
Packard, Randall M., and Paulo Gadehla. 1997. "A Land Filled with Mosquitoes: Fred L. Soper, the Rockefeller Foundation, and the Anopheles Gambiae Invasion of Brazil." *Medical Anthropology* 17 (3): 215–38.
Rockefeller Foundation. 2013. "International Health Division." Rockefeller Foundation. Accessed August 10, 2016. http://rockefeller100.org/exhibits/show/health/international-health-division.
———. 2013. "Yellow Fever." Rockefeller Foundation. Accessed August 10, 2016. http://rockefeller100.org/exhibits/show/health/yellow-fever.
Ruxin, Joshua Nalibow. 1994. "Magic Bullet: The History of Oral Rehydration Therapy." *Medical History* 38 (04): 363–97.
Starr, Paul. 1984. *The Social Transformation of American Medicine.* New York: Basic Books.
Tobbell, Dominique A. 2009. "'Who's Winning the Human Race?' Cold War as Pharmaceutical Political Strategy." *Journal of the History of Medicine and Allied Sciences* 64 (4): 429–73.
US Census Bureau, Economic Indicator Division. 2015. "U.S. Trade in Goods and Services—Balance of Payments (BOP) Basis." Washington, DC: United States Census Bureau. Accessed August 10, 2016. http://www.census.gov/foreign-trade/statistics/historical/gands.txt.

PART II

COUNTRY CASES: CHINA, JAPAN, AND SOUTH KOREA

3 Medical Education in Contemporary Mainland China

Daqing Zhang

It has been a complex and winding course for the development of medical education in mainland China since 1949. Though modern medical education in China can trace its history back to the medical school established in Canton in 1866, medical education was not officially included in the education system until 1912, when the government of the Republic of China issued the Regulation of Universities.[1] According to the regulation, medical education was to be modeled after Western patterns and the traditional model of apprenticeship was to be abolished. The curriculum adopted for medical schools contained chemistry, anatomy, and other scientific subjects. These subjects could be taught only by those who had acquired the necessary knowledge. The purpose was not to impose unfair restrictions on traditional practitioners, but to raise the standard of medical education to conform to modern international standards (Wang and Wu 1936, 160). Due to political reasons and pressure from various sources, the traditional training model was not abolished, but traditional medical schools were relabeled as training institutes (传习所) or training institutes. At the same time, many traditional medical schools revised their curriculums and added courses on scientific subjects such as anatomy, chemistry, and so on. However, due to social instability and a depressed economy, the development of medical education was insufficient to train enough medical staff as required by the needs of the people.

By 1949, there were forty-four modern medical schools and ninety traditional medical schools (Zhu 1988, 120–27), the majority of which were located in big coastal cities. Physicians who had received formal medical education numbered fewer than forty thousand, and there was not even one physician for every ten thousand people. There were only three hundred formally trained dentists and 484 pharmacists at that time. It was evident that the number of trained medical personnel could not meet the needs of the people. Thus, the government prioritized training a large number of medical personnel as soon as possible. Subsequently, over the last sixty-five years, medical education has developed and expanded significantly. Currently, there are 188 medical schools in China, from which 17,500 students graduate each year. Degree programs including bachelor's, master's, doctorate, and postgraduate medical education have been established.

While China's adoption of the teaching and practice of Western scientific medicine can be traced back to both the Qing and Republican periods, this chapter focuses specifically on the development and organization of the current system of medical education in mainland China since 1949. China's medical education system is one of the largest in the world and faces correspondingly large challenges in light of current national health care reforms, specifically matching institutional and instructional design with the goals and pace of the reforms. To review the development and current challenges of medical education in China, this chapter is organized by three chronological stages: the initial establishment of a new medical education system, the disruptive decade of the Cultural Revolution, and the current period of reconstruction and development.

Establishment of a New System in 1949

This first stage can be further subdivided into two smaller phases: recovery and establishment from 1949 to 1952 before changes to the college system and medical education reforms from 1952 to 1965.

The New Education System (1949–1952)

As of 1949, higher medical education in China had two systems that were divided along the political affiliations of opposing sides of the Chinese Civil War (1927–1949): public, private, and missionary medical schools rooted in Nationalist-held regions and medical schools in Communist areas. The Nationalist schools, which followed the Western model of medical education, were mainly located in big cities and treaty ports such as Shanghai, Guangzhou, Beijing, and Hankou. Since funds from the central and provincial governments were limited, medical students were few in number, and the length of study varied at different schools. As a result, teaching quality varied and the number of trained students was limited. Later, the Communist Party of China (CPC) established another kind of medical school to quickly train medical personnel who were urgently needed during the civil war. Although the condition of these schools had improved since 1947, they usually did not have a stable location, length of study, or curriculum. After the establishment of People's Republic of China with the Communist victory in 1949, one of the new government's main tasks was to take over medical schools from Nationalist areas and explore how to establish a new system of medical education.

At the beginning of the new Communist government, there was a severe shortage of medical personnel. Dr. Yu Yiti pointed out, "Supposing 1 physician was needed for 1,000 people, there was a shortage of 475,000 physicians.

In addition, graduates were mainly specialized in clinical medicine, and those in biomedical science and public health were very rare" (Yu 1949, 5). At this time, the central government decided to train medical personnel at two different levels: assistant doctors for county hospitals and general physicians for city hospitals (He 1950, 547–53).

At the First National Hygienic Conference, in August of 1950, the central government passed a resolution that the training of the health care professionals should be further divided into three levels to meet the differing demands for personnel in different regions: primary health workers who were trained for a short time, assistant doctors who were trained for two or three years, and physicians who were trained in medical schools for five years. The resolution indicated that the medical college should focus on training doctors in specialized subjects—surgery, pediatrics, gynecology, and so on—in order to build their competence in a clinical subject in a short period of time. The conference also passed a motion to implement a specialty-emphasis system: students should take basic medical courses in the first two years, emphasize one main clinical course in the next two years in combination with essential clinical supplementary courses, and do clinical training in the main specialty in the last year. This system shortened the training time of interns and residents from three years to one year.

In 1947, on the initiative of Wang Bin, president of China Medical University (中国医科大学), a five-year specialty-emphasis teaching system was established at the university, which cut out biomedical courses such as anatomy and physiology on the rationale that this would allow students to focus on a clinical specialty, such as surgery or pediatrics (Jin 1950, 3). The length of study for internal medicine, surgery, gynecology and obstetrics, and pediatrics was five years, with an internship in the specialized field in the last half-year. The length of study for ophthalmology, otorhinolaryngology, and dermatovenereology was four years, with an internship in the specialized field the last half-year. In public health, the length of study was four years, with a specialized internship in the last half-year. Dentistry and pharmacy programs were both four years. In the pharmacy division, there were five departments: pharmaceutics, pharmaceutical chemistry, pharmacognosy, medical laboratory science, and pharmaceutical engineering. In addition, medical schools established special two-year training programs (专修科) with an additional six-month internship for medicine, public health, and dentistry (Gao 1951, 3). Wang Bin claimed the system could train a good number of practical health care personnel as quickly as possible.

After admission, the students were assigned to different areas of study such as surgery, internal medicine, ophthalmology, and otorhinolaryngology. The proportion of students was set as 6:2:1, that is, six for surgery, two for internal medicine, and one for ophthalmology or otorhinolaryngology. Wang believed the arrangement to be in accordance with the actual demand. By 1951, 95 percent of the forty-one medical schools in China had shortened their length of study and expanded student enrollment. That year, the number of undergraduate students in medical schools around the nation was about twenty thousand, exceeding the total number of physicians who graduated in the previous sixty-nine years (*People's Daily* Editors 1951, 3).

In addition to a new emphasis on training in clinical specialties, visual teaching methods were adopted that involved the use of specimens, models, figures, animal experiments, and clinical cases. Visual teaching methods set specialty training apart from other basic courses. Teaching groups also became an important part of the new education system. The teachers in a department were divided into teaching groups according to different courses, and the teaching groups included professors, teaching assistants, and graduate students. Under the guidance of the director of the department, teaching groups conducted research on pedagogy, with the goal of improving the quality of teaching, including course instruction and curriculum design. Teaching group members attended each other's classes and provided suggestions in order to evaluate teaching capability and improve teaching performance.

The Ministry of Health (MOH) supported and promoted the new medical education model focused on training specialists and asked all of the medical schools to learn from the experience of medical schools in northeast China. However, there were also many scholars with opposing ideas who argued that the system focused on training specialist physicians could solve only the problem of the quantity of medical students, rather than address the quality of graduates and that this was not in accordance with the standard of formal medical education.

Due to the shortage of medical personnel, the central government planned to train a large number of assistant doctors in a short period of time. The main training program was for assistant doctors, which involved enrolling graduates of junior middle schools and whose length of study was two years. If there were not enough such graduates, primary school graduates were also admitted, but with the added requirement of an additional year of study. Health care and epidemic prevention were emphasized in the curriculum, and treatment was only supplementary. From 1950 to 1951, the national medical assistant schools and schools of health care had increased from twenty-three to ninety, medical assistant students increased from around twenty-six hundred to more than eighty-four hundred graduating each year. The length of study for midwives and nurses was also shortened from three years to two years. In addition, the qualification for applicants changed to needing only to have graduated from junior high school, and consequently, enrollment numbers expanded. Primary health education contained short-term training of maternal and children's health care workers (six months) and rural health workers (three months), who mainly worked in rural regions. Generally speaking, the training of primary health workers was conducted by county health centers and nursing schools. In the first half of 1951, there were over twenty-six thousand maternal and children health hygienists and more than ten thousand nurse assistants trained by this program. More than seventy thousand old-style midwives were trained in 1951.

This new medical education system helped to relieve the shortage of medical personnel, but some medical schools did not adopt it. Some people argued that this model could not provide good medical education and, thus, took an attitude of passive resistance to the new system. Others, meanwhile, thought that the shortened period of schooling would greatly reduce the quality of students. The promoters of the new system claimed that, although the period of schooling was shortened, new textbooks, new teaching groups, and new methodology could greatly increase the quality of medical education and that the so-called "regular system" did not tackle the difficult circumstances of China at that particular time. Therefore, health administrative departments fully promoted the new medical education system to cultivate more medical personnel in a short time in order to try to meet the population's demand (*People's Daily* Editors 1951, 3).

Medical Education Reforms (1952–1965)

In 1952, the Chinese government began to make comprehensive changes to the college system and in departments of higher education, modeling them on the Soviet system, and, thus, set the basic pattern of China's higher education through the latter half of twentieth century. In this pattern, the professional schools that were part of larger universities were reorganized as independent colleges (such as when the Medical School of Peking University became Beijing Medical College). For medical schools, there were two major changes. First, a general change in all institutions of higher education in 1952 reduced the number of medical schools from forty-four to thirty-one (see Table 3.1.)

Though the quantity was reduced, the scale and distribution of the colleges was more reasonable: campuses were expanded, facilities were renewed, the number of teachers was enlarged, and more students were enrolled. In 1954, there were undergraduate medical students, a great deal more than the total number of students who graduated before 1949.

The other primary policy change in medical education came in 1955 and aimed to adjust the distributions of disciplines, reaffirm prior disciplines, and steadily improve quality. According to the policy, public health and pharmaceutics departments in medical schools were reorganized. Six departments of public health were formed (at Beijing Medical College, Harbin Medical University, Shanghai First Medical College, Sichuan Medical College, Shanxi Medical College, and Central South Tongji Medical College). Two colleges (Nanjing College of Pharmacy and Shenyang College of Pharmacy) and three departments of pharmacy (at Beijing Medical College, Shanghai First Medical College, and

Table 3.1. Medical Colleges before Reorganization in 1950 and after Reorganization in 1952.

	1950	1952
1	Peking University Medical School (北京大学医学院)	Beijing Medical College (北京医学院)
2	Peking Union Medical College (北京协和医学院)	Peking Union Medical College (北京协和医学院)
3	Hebei Medical College (河北省立医学院)	Hebei Medical College (河北医学院)
4	Shanxi University Medical College (山西大学医学院)	Shanxi Medical College (山西医学院)
5	China Medical University (中国医科大学)	China Medical University (中国医科大学)
		Northeastern Pharmaceutical College (东北药学院)
6	Harbin Medical University (哈尔滨医科大学)	Harbin Medical University (哈尔滨医科大学)
7	Dalian University Medical School (大连大学医学院)	Dalian Medical College (大连医学院)
8	Cheeloo University School of Medicine (齐鲁大学医学院)	Shandong Medical College (山东医学院)
9	Shandong Provincial Medical College (山东省立医学院)	
10	Shandong University Medical School (山东大学医学院)	Qingdao Medical College (青岛医学院)
11	Nanjing University Medical School (南京大学医学院)	
12	Zhejiang University Medical School (浙江大学医学院)	Zhejiang Medical College (浙江医学院)
13	Zhejiang Provincial Medical College (浙江省立医学院)	
14	Shanghai Medical College (上海医学院)	Shanghai Medical College (上海医学院)
15	China-France University Pharmacy School (中法大学药科)	
16	St. John's University Medical School (圣约翰大学医学院)	Shanghai Second Medical College (上海第二医学院)
17	University Medical School (震旦大学医学院)	
18	Tongde Medical College (同德医学院)	
19	Shanghai Dentist Special School (上海牙医专科学院)	
20	Southeastern Medical College (东南医学院)	Anhui Medical College (安徽医学院)
21	Jiangsu Medical College (江苏医学院)	Nanjing Medical College (南京医学院)

22	Eastern China Pharmacy School (华东药学专科学校)	Eastern China Pharmaceutical College (华东药学院)
23	Soochow University Pharmacy School (东吴大学药学专修科)	
24	Fujian Provincial Medical College (福建省立医学院)	Fujian Medical College (福建医学院)
25	Hunan-Yale Medical College (湘雅医学院)	Hunan Medical College (湖南医学院)
26	North Jiangsu Medical College (苏北医学院)	Nantong Medical College (南通医学院)
27	Central China Medical College (华中医学院)	Jiangxi Medical College (江西医学院)
28	Jiangxi Provincial Medical College (江西省立医学专科学校)	
29	Henan University Medical College (河南大学医学院)	Henan Medical College (河南医学院)
30	Tongji University Medical School (同济大学医学院)	Wuhan Medical College (武汉医学院)
31	Wuhan University Medical School (武汉大学医学院)	
32	Hubei Provincial Medical College (湖北省立医学院)	Hubei Medical College (湖北医学院)
33	Guangxi Provincial Medical College (广西省立医学院)	Guangxi Medical College (广西医学院)
34	Sun Yat-Sen University Medical School (中山大学医学院)	Zhongshan Medical College (中山医学院)
35	Lingnan University Medical School (岭南大学医学院)	
36	Guangdong Guanghua Medical College (广东光华医学院)	
37	Northwestern University Medical School (西北大学医学院)	Xian Medical College (西安医学院)
38	Lanzhou University Medical School (兰州大学医学院)	Lanzhou Medical College (兰州医学院)
39	University Medical School (华西协和大学医学院)	Sichuan Medical College (四川医学院)
40	Chongqing University Medical School (重庆大学医学院)	
41	Guiyang Medical College (贵阳医学院)	Guiyang Medical College (贵阳医学院)
42	Yunnan University Medical School (云南大学医学院)	Yunnan Medical College (云南医学院)
43	Changchun Military Medical College (长春军医大学)	China People's Liberation Army Third Military Medical College (中国人民解放军第三军医大学)
44	China People's Liberation Army Tianjin Military Medical College (中国人民解放军天津军医大学)	China People's Liberation Army First Military Medical College (中国人民解放军第一军医大学)

Sichuan Medical College) were also formed. In this change, forensic medicine was dropped as a major with the reasoning that, with the development of socialism and the elimination of social class, enemies of the people would be gradually wiped out and forensic medicine would no longer be needed (Zhu and Zhang 1990, 10).

Following systematic changes in colleges and departments, the Ministry of Education demanded that the institutions of higher education translate and compile Soviet teaching materials and the Ministry of Health authorized some institutions to translate Soviet textbooks and teaching programs in medicine and pharmacy. By 1955, twenty-four Soviet medical textbooks and ten practical handbooks were published. The Chinese government also invited Soviet medical experts. At first, all the medical experts were hosted at Beijing Medical College and taught teachers' training classes that enrolled and trained crucial faculty from medical colleges and universities across China. In some clinical majors, the Soviet experts were excellent, but this was not always the case in biomedical sciences. For this reason, teachers who had been educated in medicine in Europe or America found certain Soviet experts lacking. Even so, Soviet medicine impacted the medical educational system in China. Examples of this include the formation of public health departments and epidemic prevention stations, the promotion of Kaiipob's three-center educational method (class center, teacher center, and textbook center), and advocacy and teaching of Pavlovian theories. The Soviet system emphasized the training of practical ability in clinical medicine and neglected basic theories in biology and biomedicine, such as genetics and cellular pathology. Ironically, Virchow's theory of cellular pathology and Morgan's theory of genetics were criticized as the theories of the bourgeoisie.

In 1954, the Ministry of Higher Education and the Ministry of Health held the first joint National Higher Medical Education Conference. At the conference, college-level medical education became the policy priority instead of middle-level medical education. The Ministry of Education and the Ministry of Health jointly formulated a scheme for the length of study and standards for teaching schedules. The conference also included discussion regarding how Chinese medicine should enter into higher medical education. The conference urged all medical colleges to gradually set up courses in Chinese medicine, a recommendation proposed by Mao Zedong. In the early 1950s, He Cheng, chief of the Central Ministry of Health believed that the development of modern medicine would replace Chinese medicine and that most of the Chinese-medicine physicians were lacking in medical knowledge and in need of further education. When the Ministry of Health announced a plan for doctors of Chinese medicine to study Western medicine at continuation schools, doctors of Chinese medicine pushed back.

Aware of the complaints of doctors of Chinese medicine, Mao Zedong, Liu Shaoqi, and Zhou Enlai stated that Chinese medicine was a splendid cultural heritage and that it should be further explored and improved. "Traditional Chinese Medicine has a history of thousands of years," said an editorial in the *People's Daily* of October 20, 1954. "It has rich content and valuable clinical experience, playing an important role in fighting against diseases over the past generations. It is a glorious task for medical personnel to inherit and promote this cultural heritage, to learn its theory and practice earnestly, to sort and summarize by a scientific method, to improve its academic and medical levels, and to make it more effective to serve the people" (*People Daily*, Editors 1954, 1).

While requiring courses on Chinese medicine in medical colleges and universities, the central government developed a plan to establish four colleges of Chinese medicine and suggested that one should be established in every direction, with one each in the eastern, western, northern, and southern parts of China. In 1956, colleges of Chinese medicine were officially established in Beijing, Shanghai, Guangzhou, and Chengdu. Gradually, traditional Chinese medicine (TCM) colleges or departments in other provinces and cities were also established. In spite of differences of opinion regarding what should constitute an appropriate curriculum, such as how to strike a balance between Western medicine and TCM and what should be the sequence of learning them, Chinese medicine was finally officially incorporated into the higher education system under the direct auspices of the central government.

There had always been different opinions regarding the length of schooling for medical education, and some officers and scholars from the Ministries of Health and Education favored a single standard. In 1957, the Ministry of Health and the Ministry Education proposed that some colleges and universities could establish six-year programs for training excellent medical students. Due to the movement of the Great Leap Forward, which began in 1958, the number of Chinese medical colleges abruptly increased from 37 to 204 in only a year's time. This kind of expansion went beyond the managerial ability of existing administrations, and the teaching conditions also soon caused a series of difficulties such as lack of teachers and equipment and decline in the quality of teaching.

In 1960, the central government began to correct the policy of expanding the medical schools recklessly. A large number of unqualified colleges were closed, and the number was reduced to eighty-five. In 1962, the Ministry of Health and the Ministry of Education issued the "Notice about changing the length of schooling in higher medical colleges and universities" (J. Zhang 1982, 320–21). Then, major medical colleges and universities adopted a system of longer length of schooling because medical schools had too many courses and the longer length would reduce the burden students had each term. Another reason for prolonging the length of schooling was to strengthen the training in basic theory, knowledge, and skills, as well as to improve the quality of teaching. However, the policy of extending schooling length was criticized by Mao Zedong. In 1964, he pointed out at the Spring Festival Forum that "the length of schooling should be shortened and the courses should be simplified" (Mao 1967, 72). As a result, the reform of longer length of schooling was revoked in twenty-one colleges and universities, such as Beijing Second Medical College, Zhejiang Medical University, and Harbin Medical University. Soon after that, the Ministry of Health issued a notice requiring medical colleges and universities to simplify the content of their teaching and to improve teaching methods, thereby relieving the burden on students and improving the quality of foreign language teaching, but the six-year medical length of schooling for medical majors did not change.

Early in 1965, Mao Zedong again criticized the health care system and medical education. He stated that the health care delivery system did not satisfactorily meet the needs of rural communities and did not serve the broad masses of peasants. He stated that medical education should be reformed and that the emphasis of medical and health care work should be in rural areas. On January 20, 1965, the Ministry of Health reported that fifteen medical colleges had started medical programs three years in length for the purpose of training rural doctors. In August, the Ministry of Health held the National Higher Medical Education Conference in Beidaihe and proposed that higher medical education must implement the policy of "walking on two legs" to cultivate medical and health personnel who were greater, faster, and thriftier. Programs with both long and short durations of schooling should coexist, but shorter should be the main form. Most medical junior colleges should be established in rural areas, and students should be enrolled from communes and return to communes after graduation as part of the "half-peasant, half-student" system. Developed medical schools should be encouraged to expand into rural regions and train health workers at the local level. The conference made the resolution to change the length of schooling for medical programs from six years to five years, and pharmacy programs from five years to four years (*People's Daily* Editors 1965, 1).

The Cultural Revolution (1966–1976)

Generally speaking, the entire educational system in China was disrupted by the Cultural Revolution. For four years, from 1966 to 1970, medical education ground to a halt. Normal teaching activities at medical schools were stopped, and no students were enrolled. By 1968, Mao Zedong proposed that universities resume their activities but that the length of schooling be shortened and the education model be changed in order to adapt the needs of the health of the people. After 1970, medical colleges and universities opened again and a plan was adopted that both shortened the length of schooling and admitted students from varied educational backgrounds. The length of schooling for medical majors was shortened from five years to three years, and the length of schooling for pharmaceutical majors was shortened from four years to two years. Admitted students were from worker, peasant, and soldier backgrounds whose educational levels varied considerably from high school graduate to primary school graduate. "Open-door education" and "students coming from the communes and returning to the communes after graduation" were policies advocated during this period.

In the second phase, although medical education began to recover gradually, it was fashioned to participate in a politically motivated "Medical Education Revolution." For example, the government mandated that medical colleges service rural regions and many teachers and even some medical colleges were moved to the countryside. During this period, teaching in classrooms and city hospitals, and even the use of foreign medical equipment in clinical practice, were often criticized as cut off from real society and not serving peasants. The traditional curriculum—from anatomy, physiology, and other basic medical courses to clinical training—was criticized as a Western capitalistic training model that needed to be changed completely. During their three years of study, these worker, peasant, and soldier students were required to attend political activities on a regular basis, as well as be involved in industrial and agricultural production and military training. Actually, they spent a very limited amount of time on their study of medical knowledge and training for clinical practice. Therefore, physicians who graduated during this period were not well-equipped to provide adequate medical services.

Although higher medical education gradually recovered under the slogan of starting an "education revolution," what constituted good medical education became a controversial issue. Ever since Western medicine was introduced into China, there has always existed sharp disagreement on how to deal with the two systems, Chinese medicine and Western medicine. During the period of the original Republic of China, despite resistance from traditional medical practitioners, Chinese medicine was excluded from the formal medical education system. After the founding of the People's Republic of China, Chinese medicine was not included in the higher medical education system until 1956. During the Cultural Revolution, under the influence of "creating unified new medicine in China" and the ideology of revolution in education, some colleges and universities of Chinese medicine and Western medicine were merged and "new medical colleges" were established, but by the end of the decade, these institutions of "new medicine" were separated back into medical colleges of either Western medicine or TCM (see Table 3.2).

Under the influence of political campaigns, the merging of colleges and universities was unreasonable academically and could be not broadly supported by faculty and administrators. Many people questioned what was new in these "universities of new medicine." Premier Zhou Enlai also showed deep concern about the mergers, saying, "The combination of Chinese medicine and Western medicine is right, but are we ready to merge the colleges and universities of Western and Chinese medicine? If we don't have the proper conditions, it can be postponed" (Zhu and Zhang 1990, 147). This practice of merging colleges later proved that

Table 3.2. Medical Colleges before, during, and after Merger of Western and Traditional Chinese Medical Colleges.

Medical Colleges Before Merger and After Separation	Merged Institutions, Including Years of Merger
Hebei Medical College Tianjin College of Traditional Chinese Medicine	Hebei University of New Medicine (1970–1979)
Nanjing Medical College Nanjing College of Traditional Chinese Medicine	Jiangsu College of New Medicine (1970–1979)
Zhejiang Medical College Zhejiang College of Traditional Chinese Medicine	Zhejiang Medical University (1970–1974)
Anhui Medical College Anhui College of Traditional Chinese Medicine	Anhui Medical College (1970–1975)
Jilin Medical University Changchun College of Traditional Chinese Medicine	Jilin Medical University (1970–1978)
Fujian Medical College Fujian College of Traditional Chinese Medicine	Fujian Medical University (1969–1978)
Shandong Medical College Shandong College of Traditional Chinese Medicine	Shandong Medical College (1970–1975)
Jiangxi Medical College Jiangxi College of Traditional Chinese Medicine	Jiangxi Medical University (1969–1972)

this kind of political interference neither brought development opportunities to the merged schools nor created a new mode of operating schools. Instead, owing to changes in personnel and organization, it had adverse effects. For example, at these universities of new medicine, the length of schooling was compressed to only three years and yet students were required to learn both modern medicine and traditional Chinese medicine. The result was that students could not master both medical knowledge systems because of the limited amount of study time. Therefore, the model of so-called "new medicine universities" proved unsuccessful after just a few years, and those universities were divided into independent, separate medical colleges.

Reconstruction and Development (1977–Present)

By October 1976, with the downfall of the "Gang of Four," China's medical education entered into a period of restoration and reconstruction. Due to economic growth, medical education went through a stage of great and rapid development that was accompanied by a rising demand for health care. Since China's economic reforms and opening-up, which began in 1978, China's medical colleges have increasingly cooperated with foreign medical schools. This exchange in higher medical education has led to the teaching of new medical theories, new teaching methods, and new patterns in education aiming to cultivate qualified medical professionals to address the health conditions in the nation, as well as stay on top of global medical trends. This period can be divided into two stages: reconstruction (1977–1993) and development (1993–present).

Reconstruction (1977–1993)

Since the National College Entrance Examination (*gaokao*) was restored in 1977, the Ministries of Education and Health have issued a series of relevant rules and regulations about medical education and teaching in medical schools. In 1978, postgraduate enrollment was restored and the classification of disciplines and degree-granting institutions in medicine was confirmed, constituting a tiered medical education system including undergraduate and postgraduate training (i.e., bachelor's, master's, and doctorate in a three-tiered system). In June 1980, the Ministries of Education and Health jointly convened the National Conference on Medical Education, in which past experiences and lessons were reviewed and summarized and questions concerning how to elevate teaching quality, how to strengthen faculty development, how to raise the quality of teaching material, and how to improve teaching management were also discussed. The Plan for Development of China's Higher Medical Education and The Idea about Setting and Adjustment of Disciplines in Medical School were revised at the conference and established a basic framework for the training of medical and pharmaceutical professionals.

China is a huge country geographically, demographically, and ethnically, and, consequently, the level of economic development and the level of medical science and technology vary enormously by region. The need for health care services follows the same basic pattern, as there still exist deficiencies in medical personnel in remote and rural areas and ethnic minority areas. Since the 1980s, the government has intended to further adjust the regional distribution of medical training. In 1983, the Ministry of Health and the State Ethnic Affairs Commission jointly convened the National Health Conference for Ethnic Minorities and formulated a series of blueprints, such as The Plan for Training Minority Medical Professionals. Thereafter, four ethnic minority colleges set up premed courses and it became compulsory for key medical universities in Beijing, Shanghai, Guangzhou, and other big cities to enroll minority students from the five autonomous regions, including Guangxi, Inner Mongolia, Ningxia, Xinjiang, and Tibet.

Along with economic reform and socioeconomic transformation, the Chinese medical system has been on a mission for further reform. However, in the field of health care management, China is still suffering from a lack of elite professionals. In modern society, health care is not simply about the prevention and treatment of disease, but also a set of complex institutional arrangements—including the distribution of health resources and social welfare—that motivates a number of specialists in medicine, business, and hospital management. In 1982, the Ministry of Health established facilities for the training of medical professionals in seven medical schools, including Beijing Medical College, which later developed an undergraduate program of health care management. In 1984, the Ministry of Health launched a project to train the heads of health and sanitary bureaus of provinces and deans of medical schools all over the country with the intention of finishing rotational training of major directors in the health sector within three years. This project played an important and active role in providing these officials in charge of health care management and medical education with the latest knowledge and practices in medical education and health care-related fields in terms of scope of knowledge and scientific management methodologies.

In 1979, Deng Xiaoping proposed focusing on developing the education of science and technology as a top priority. Programs with a foreign-language emphasis for students (a six-year system) were set up in ten medical colleges, including Beijing Medical College, in order to train excellent students and send them to study abroad. The aim of the program was to cultivate talents for future use. In the same year, Dr. Patrick Ongley, president of the China Medical Board (CMB), and a few CMB trustees visited China after its reopening to the West. This marked CMB's return to China after leaving in 1949 and one of the first visits to China by an American foundation since the nation's opening up. In his report to CMB's trustees, Dr. Ongley pointed out that the Chinese schools' greatest needs at the time included the development of more adequate basic science departments and the training of future research workers. He advised that a wise use of funds would be in the fields of medical education and research. He suggested that CMB should aid several schools rather than concentrate all its efforts in one school, as it had done previously when it concentrated its funding on the Peking Union Medical College from 1914 to 1950. The exponential effects of funding a small, select group of major schools would make a greater contribution than support of any one school (Norris 2003, 112–15). CMB's strategies for medical education have had a long history of success, and it has played an important role in establishing modern medical education in China (D. Zhang 2009, 137–55). CMB provided vital support for medical education from the very beginning of China's economic reforms, offering much needed financial support for the development of medical education and human resources before China's economy took off. CMB facilitated communication and interconnectedness between China and the West in the field of medical education and played an important role in the introduction of new teaching methods and medical education reforms. Through its capacity-building efforts, its impact is even greater. Medical schools and scholars that have benefited from CMB have taken on leadership roles in Chinese medical education reforms. CMB's contributions to the development of medical education in China and other countries in East Asia are discussed in more detail in chapter 1 of this volume.

Starting in the opening up period, the Chinese government also engaged in international developments in medical education. Due to the demand for better health care services, stricter standards were put in place for a new generation of health care professionals. When a biopsychosocial medical model was introduced into China in the 1980s, this notion in particular had a significant impact in bringing about medical education reforms. Various disciplines in the humanities and the social sciences became incorporated into medical education curriculums, including such subjects as medical psychology, medical ethics, medical philosophy, and health economics.

In 1988, a Chinese delegation attended the Conference of the World Federation for Medical Education (WFME). The Edinburgh Declaration set forth the recommendations of the conference, calling for reforms in medical education to take extensive and effective actions to achieve health for all by the year 2000. The Declaration played an important role in the reform of medical education and professional training in China.

Development (1993–Present)

The year 1993 is considered a turning point for China's higher education, as this was the year when the *Outline of Reform and Development of China's Education* was published by the central government. It suggested that "education development should be oriented to modernization, the world and the future; the reform and development of education should be secured; this is in order to create a more highly skilled workforce, to be committed to fostering human resources, and to constitute an education system which is adapted to the socialist market economic system and political, science and technology reforms." As the *Outline* stated, "in order to take on the challenges of the new technological revolution, the strength of central and local sectors should be gathered to support more or less 100 key universities and a group of key disciplines and specialties, with the aim of gaining global prominence in educational quality, scientific research and educational management" (Zhonggong Zhongyang Guowuyuan Yinfa 1993, 2).

While the implementation of the *Outline* provided an impetus for the development of Chinese medical education, pressure for reform was imposed all along. First of all, some select medical schools were included in the Project 211 University List (for instance, Beijing Medical University being merged into Peking

University and Shanghai Medical University into Fudan University) and obtained powerful assistance from the government in terms of human resources, funding, and construction, which provided opportunities and security for the development of medical education. Second, given the economic system, specific reform measures were raised—for example, the expansion of student enrollment—which led to an increase in the number of students in medical schools. It is estimated that there was a fourfold increase in enrollment in only ten years, with the population of students increasing from 66,877 in 1993 to 257,681 in 2003. Third, medical graduates were granted the freedom to search for jobs by and for themselves, although they soon began to feel the pressure and difficulty of finding jobs on their own. There is an imbalanced relationship between employment opportunities for medical graduates and people's health care needs, as most graduates prefer to work at large-scale hospitals in medium- and large-sized cities, rather than in rural, remote areas or at community hospitals where, paradoxically, the need for health care professionals is far greater.

By the late 1990s, although the number of medical colleges and universities, the scale of enrollment, and the number of specialties had increased, the medical curriculum had been changed by the introduction of the bio-psycho-socio-medical patterns. According to the statistical data reported in the *Curriculum Guide for Chinese Medical Universities and Colleges* (1998), almost all the medical schools had similar educational objectives and teaching requirements for clinical medicine. The core courses were basic and clinical medicine. All curriculum design was discipline-centered, with 46 percent of medical schools having elective courses, of which 31 percent were within areas related to the humanities and social sciences. The ratio of required versus elective courses was roughly three to one. For all schools, the educational process was divided into three stages: general education courses, medical sciences courses, and clinical specialist courses. It has been noted that early exposure to clinical practice was arranged in a few cases. The primary teaching method was theoretical teaching by means of teacher-centered lectures and group-based experiments through internships (Jiaoyubu Gaodeng Jiaoyu Si 1998).

The Chinese medical community is aware that China's medical education is behind most industrialized countries and has endeavored to alter the situation. They suggest that the nation's medical education should follow the trend of globalization. Drawing on advances in medical education, many medical universities have been constantly working on adjusting their educational strategy since the beginning of the twenty-first century. Some research sponsored by the Ministry of Education has recommended that international standards should be applied to China's medical education scheme so as to improve and ensure the quality of medical education. Some priorities are the optimization of course structure, active exploration into integrated courses, updating teaching content, enhancement of cutting-edge courses, highlighting and strengthening students' innovation, creativity, and practical ability, and overall quality. At the same time, it has also been recognized that training health care workers needed in rural areas should be a priority, considering the deficiency of medical personnel in such areas (D. Wang 2005, 1–4). In May 2002, commissioned by the Western Pacific Regional Office and the Ministries of Education and Health, Peking University Health Science Center and the National Institute of Higher Medical Education jointly convened a "Symposium on International Standards of Medical Education," which aimed to promote the reform and further development of Chinese medical education through the introduction and pilot study of two international standards of medical education: the International Standards in Basic Medical Education by WFME (1999) and the WHO Guidelines for Quality Assurance of Basic Medical Education in the Western Pacific Region by WHO-WPRO (2001). Meanwhile, with the endorsement of CMB and the Institute for International Medical Education, research on "Global Minimum Essential Requirements in Medical Education" was carried out at eight medical universities, including Peking University Health Science Center, Fudan University Shanghai Medical College, and Chinese Medical University. Based on the results of this research, in early 2003, the Ministry of Education officially approved the project of a "Study on the Quality Assurance System of Medical Education," with the objectives of creating localized medical education standards, constructing a Medical Education Accreditation System of China with reference to relevant international standards, and optimizing the medical education assurance system, i.e., the Chinese Undergraduate Medical Education Standards.

Current Challenges

In December 2011, Chen Zhu, former Minister of Health, pointed out at the National Medical Education Reform Conference that the training of medical and health personnel in particular lags behind other aspects of health care system reform. Though student enrollment in medical schools has rapidly increased since 1999, the quality and quantity of graduates have not satisfied the demand for medical care services, especially in rural areas.

Medical education in China is facing great challenges, including its neglect of the humanities and social sciences in medical curriculums and the fact that it is producing more research scientists than skilled clinical doctors. The reform of medical education should follow the regular pattern of medical education. Firstly, the training of clinicians should be geared toward the mastery of both theoretical knowledge and practical skills. Each one of the three stages of medical education should have different focuses: 1) college education imparts theoretical knowledge through training in the basic sciences, assisted by clinical practice; 2) postgraduate study teaches practical skills, implemented by standardized training of residents; and 3) continuing education ensures that practicing physicians are kept up to date with current practices and medical developments.

Currently, there is a human resource allocation problem in that there is a mismatch between college education and hospital requirements, a lack of a connection between college education and continuing education, and an imperfect coordination system between education and health authorities, all of which hinder improvements in health care service. Medical education in China does not have a unified system. Currently, there are three-year, five-year, seven-year, and eight-year programs (which consist of "5+3" or "4+4").[2] The training of medical graduate students tends to emphasize scientific research rather than clinical practice. For this reason, clinical training is weak, rendering medical graduates unable to meet clinical requirements, especially the shortage of general practitioners eligible for the treatment of common diseases. The evaluation of doctors is based on journal publications rather than clinical skills, which leads to an overemphasis on research and distracts doctors' attention away from the diagnosis and treatment of patients.

The Achilles' heel of Chinese medical education is its neglect of the humanities and social sciences. In China, medicine has been considered a natural science instead of a discipline studied for the sake of humanity. Patient-doctor conflicts have been attributed to the doctors' inadequate ethical and legal conscience and weak interpersonal communication ability. The focus on social and ethical aspects of medical education has increasingly attracted attention in China. Many medical universities have set up courses in medical ethics and law, as well as in patient-doctor communication. In 2013, the Ministry of Education created a Steering Committee for courses on humanities in medical colleges and universities (earlier, a sub-committee was founded under the rubric of a basic medical education committee). In addition, less conspicuous courses emphasizing humaneness and related social practices are also being implemented.

China has the largest medical education system in the world. The number of students enrolled in medical schools was up to 1.86 million in 2010. Although medical education in China has progressed considerably over the past thirty years, the system needs further reform. For instance, as the lengths of degree programs have become longer and longer, medical degrees have become more and more specialized, yet clinical internships have become more and more brief. Heavy emphasis is placed on theory and textbook knowledge, while skills and practice are put to the side. Medical education should be an integrated educational process consisting of college, postgraduate education, and continuous education. Moreover, the development of individual potential has been neglected during the training of general practitioners and residents. Under the current orientation of the economic market, there are not enough qualified medical workers in rural or remote areas, while hospitals in midsized or large cities do not have sufficient capacity for all the medical graduates who would like to work there. Therefore, many medical personnel end up quitting and seeking other jobs, resulting in a huge brain drain. In the current situation, the overall demand for medical professionals has not been met and structural imbalances remain. There appears to be an oversupply of medical graduates, but the quality of medical professionals varies greatly, especially given the lack of unifying standards for training residents (Yang 2008, 13).

Another predicament is how to attract the best students. In most countries, the best students enroll in medical universities because doctors generally enjoy the advantages of higher social status and stable and substantial income. However, for the most talented Chinese students, even the best medical university is not the top option. In addition, many parents, including those who are doctors, do not want their children to choose medicine for their future career. This is because of the rising tensions between patients and doctors in recent years, as is evidenced by increasing violence in medical encounters, in which health personnel often become the victims. One doctor relates, "When I entered the medical profession years ago, I was filled with heartfelt pride and overwhelming professional achievement. However, the drama of hospital violence has become so frequent, which reflects the complete collapse of basic trust in the patient-doctor relationship. This is not merely a pity for the doctor, but also a source of shame for society" (Liu 2013, 20–21).

Conclusion

There are three kinds of tensions that have driven the development of medical education in contemporary China. The first is the tension between politics and medicine. From the emphasis on training specialists in the Soviet model in the 1950s, to the disruptive education revolution in the 1970s, and then to the standardization of universities in the 1990s, the evolution of medical education in China occurred under a series of political interventions, rather than as an independent progress consisting of adaptations to the social and economic environment. One advantage of this is that the government can adjust the medical education system directly and quickly, including promoting more equitable distribution of medical personnel and adjusting the emphasis of health work. But the negative effects seem to be greater—for instance, when medical education policy changes without consideration of the long-term effects. The changes in the medical education system often took place in parallel to political changes that did not follow the logic of a development in medical education. In the 1950s, China adopted Soviet-style education under an all-encompassing political view. It denied the concept of higher education and rejected beneficial academic traditions from Europe and America (and ejected their institutions from the People's Republic of China), and it abandoned general education for undergraduates.

School management also changed from diversification to centralization. This kind of Soviet model led to an emphasis on skills training and specialization, leading to the separation of humanities and science education and caused distortions in students' knowledge and limitations in their thoughts. In particular, the Chinese government mainly considered short-term needs and sought quick successes, and for this reason, courses not directly related to practical skills were canceled, leading to a lack of humanism. Politically bound education reached its climax during the Cultural Revolution, during which admission standards for medical students, curriculum standards, and standards for length of schooling all served short-term political demand. After China's economic reforms, political intervention into medical education was reduced significantly, but infractions of the rules of medical education still existed, especially in the standards for length of schooling and in the arbitrary merging of universities.

The second type of tension is that between tradition and modernity. In the process of the modernization of TCM, it has always been controversial whether it should be included in the medical education system. The establishment of Chinese medical colleges in the middle of the 1950s marked the formal entrance of Chinese medicine into the system of higher medical education. However, even today, there is still doubt of the value of Chinese medical colleges and universities, while some in TCM circles hold the view that Chinese medical education should return to the traditional tutorial system, which is thought to be conducive to the inheritance of the TCM tradition. Developing traditional medicine, promoting its modernization, and creating a "new medicine" has been a national aspiration in terms of Chinese cultural inheritance. However, Chinese medical colleges and Western medical colleges, which were merged under political pressure during the Cultural Revolution, separated soon thereafter, indicating that there are internal contradictions between TCM and Western medicine that cannot be easily solved. Even to this day, although Chinese and Western medical colleges and universities operate independently from one another, modern medical courses have been integrated into the TCM educational system and there are majors that integrate Chinese and Western medicine, yet these remain controversial.

The third tension is that between medical elitism and populism. A debate has long existed about whether medicine should focus on the cultivation of practical personnel, such as general practitioners and primary health workers, or of advanced elites, such as cardiovascular surgeons and gastroenterological specialists. At the beginning of the founding of the People's Republic of China, due to the urgent need for medical staff, the mainstream opinion was to train practical personnel. Later, normalized and advanced medical education requiring longer length of schooling became the norm. In the middle of the 1960s, Mao Zedong criticized this system because it required many years to complete, so the length of schooling was shortened. At this time, workers, peasants, and soldiers were admitted to colleges. After China's economic reforms, the longer length of schooling resumed. The contradictions in contemporary medical reform also point to talent cultivation. The eight-year clinical doctoral education had been criticized to the extent that it was considered to be not as good as the five-year program because of its deficiency in clinical practice and relevant skills. The eight-year length of schooling has now become a "5 + 3" system, returning to five years of formal education combined with residency training. At the same time, the three-year junior training system for rural physicians has also been questioned. Critics point out that there is no intrinsic reason why the level of medical service in rural areas should be lower than that in urban areas.

The history of medical education in contemporary China is a rich seam to mine, full of examples of interesting and controversial practices and widespread reevaluation of the aims of medicine. There is more to be done and more to be learned from the past. It remains a huge challenge to envisage how medical education and the medical profession can cope with a series of dilemmas in health care reform. Medical education needs to be clear about its role in training respectable doctors who are educated to mobilize their knowledge for the right purposes, doctors who engage in critical reasoning and ethical conduct so that they are competent and ready "to participate in patient-centered and population-centered health systems as members of locally responsive and globally connected teams" (Frenk et al. 2010, 1923–58).

Notes

1. The Regulation of Universities is a regulation for managing universities and colleges, including the category of the university, the length of schooling, and the standards for entrance into the university.

2. The three-year system is for students in junior colleges and provides no degrees. The five-year system is for students to obtain a medical bachelor's degree. The seven-year system is for students to obtain a medical master's degree. The eight-year system is for students to become a doctor.

References

Frenk, Julio, Lincoln Chen, Zulfiqar A. Bhutta, Jordan Cohen, Nigel Crisp, Timothy Evans, Harvey Fineberg, Patricia Garcia, Yang Ke, Patrick Kelley, Barry Kistnasamy, Afaf Meleis, David Naylor, Ariel Pablos-Mendez, Srinath Reddy, Susan Scrimshaw, Jaime Sepulveda, David Serwadda, and Huda Zurayk. 2010. "Health Professionals for a New Century: Transforming Education to Strengthen Health Systems in an Interdependent World." *The Lancet* 376: 1923–58.

Gao, Chang'guo [高昌国]. 1951. "新中国的医学教育制度 [Xin Zhongguode Yixue Jiaoyu Zhidu] [The Medical Education System in New China]." 人民日报 [*Renmin Ribao*] [*People's Daily*], December 2.

He, Cheng [贺诚]. 1950. "中央人民政府卫生部贺诚副部长 在第一届全国卫生会议上的总结报告 [Zhongyang Renmin Zhengfu Weishengbu He Cheng Fubuzhang Zai Diyi Jie Quan Guo Weisheng Huiyi Shangde Zongjie Baogao] [Final Report on the First National Public Health Conference by Vice Health Minister He Cheng]." 中华新医学报 *Zhonghua Xin Yixue Bao* [*Journal of New Medicine in China*] 1 (8): 547–53.

Jiaoyubu Gaodeng Jiaoyu Si [教育部高等教育司] [Ministry of Education Higher Education Department]. 1998. 中国高等医学院校课程指南 [*Zhongguo Gaodeng Yixue Yuanxiao Kecheng Zhinan*] [*China Higher Education Medical School Course Guidebook*]. Beijing: 中国中医药出版社 [Zhongguo Zhongyi Yao Chubanshe] [China Press of Traditional Chinese Medicine].

Jin, Feng [金凤]. 1950. "东北新型的医学教育 [Dongbei Xinxingde Yixue Jiaoyu] [New Medical Education in the Northeast]." 人民日报 [*Renmin Ribao*] [*People's Daily*], June 10.

Liu, Hong [刘宏]. 2013. "莫让医者之殇成社会之痛 [Mo Rang Yizhe Zhi Shang Cheng Shehui Zhi Tong] [Do Not Let the Death of Doctors Become the Pain of Society]." 中国卫生人才 [*Zhongguo Weisheng Rencai*] [*China Public Health Personnel*] 12: 20–21.

Mao, Zedong [毛泽东]. 1967. "春节谈话 [Chunjie Tanhua Jiyao] [Remarks at the Spring Festival]." 毛泽东思想万岁 [*Mao Zedong Sixiang Wansui*] [*Long Live the Mao Zedong Ideology*]. Accessed August 9, 2016. http://www.marxists.org/chinese/PDF/08/01210804.pdf.

Norris, Laurie. 2003. *The China Medical Board: 50 Years of Programs, Partnerships, and Progress, 1950–2000*. New York: China Medical Board of New York.

People's Daily Editors [人民日报社论]. 1951. "全国推行新医学教育制度获得成绩 [Quan Guo Tuixing Xin Yixue Jiaoyu Zhidu Huode Chengji] [Achievements of Promoting the New Medical Education System in China]." 人民日报 [*Renmin Ribao*] [*People's Daily*], November 3.

———. 1954. "贯彻对待中医的正确政策 [Guanche Duidai Zhongyide Zhengque Zhengce] [Implementing Correct Policies about Traditional Chinese Medicine]." 人民日报 [*Renmin Ribao*] [*People's Daily*], October 20.

———. 1965. "全国高等医学教育会议确定面向农村办学,培养为农民服务的白求恩式医务人员,打破各种框框, 积极稳妥地改革学制、教学内容和教学方法 [Quan Guo Gaodeng Yixue Jiaoyu Huiyi Queding Mianxiang Nongcun Banxue, Peiyang Wei Nongmin Fuwude Baiqiuenshi Yiwu Renyuan, Dapo Gezhong Kuangkuang, Jiji Wentuode Gaige Xuezhi, Jiaoxue Neirong He Jiaoxue Fangfa] [The National Higher Medical Education Conference Confirms the Decision to Run Schools for Rural Areas, Cultivate Bethune-like Medical Personnel to Serve Peasants, to Break Through Every Sort of Limitation, and to Actively and Dependably Reform the Length of Schooling, as well as Educational Content and Methods of Teaching]." 人民日报 [*Renmin Ribao*] [*People's Daily*], September 8.

Wang, Debing [王德炳]. 2005. "中国高等医学教育管理体制和学制学位改革研究总体报告 [Zhongguo Gaodeng Yixue Jiaoyu Guanli Tizhi He Xuezhi Xueli Gaige Yanjiu Zongti Baogao] [Summary Report on Research on Reforming China's Higher Medical Education Administrative Systems and Length of Schooling for Academic Degrees]." *Yixue Jiaoyu* 医学教育 (*Medical Education*) 6: 1–4.

Wang, Jimin [王吉民] and Wu Liande [伍连德]. 1936. 中国医史 [*Zhongguo Yishi*][*History of Chinese Medicine*]. Shanghai: 检疫管理处 [Jianyi Guanlichu] [National Quarantine Service].

Yang, Mingfang [杨明方]. 2008. "学制越来越长, 学历越来越高, 实习越来越短, 医学教育'发育'不全 [Xuezhi Yue Lai Yue Chang, Xueli Yue Lai Yue Gao, Shixi Yue Lai Yue Duan, Yixue Jiaoyu 'Fayu' Bu Quan] [The Length of Schooling Becomes Longer and Longer, Academic Qualifications Get Higher and Higher, Practice Gets Shorter and Shorter, Medical Education 'Development' is Not Complete]." 人民日报 [Renmin Ribao] [People's Daily], April 17.

Yu, Yiti [余贻侗]. 1949. "医学的政治性 [Yixuede Zhengzhixing] [The Political Nature of Medicine]. 人民日报 [Renmin Ribao] [People's Daily], October 20.

Zhang, Daqing [张大庆]. 2009. "中国现代医学初建时期的布局:洛克菲勒基金会的影响 [Zhongguo Xiandai Yixue Chu Jian Shiqide Buju: Luokefeile Jijinhuide Yingxiang] [Mapping Modern Medicine in China: Impact of the Rockefeller Foundation]." 自然科学史研究 [Ziran Kexue Shi Yanjiu] [Studies in the History of Natural Sciences] 28 (2): 137–55.

Zhang, Jian [张健], ed. 1982. 中国教育年鉴: 1949-1981 [Zhongguo Jiaoyu Nianjian: 1949–1981] [Chinese Education Almanac: 1949–1981]. Beijing: 中国大百科全书出版社 [Zhongguo Da Baikequanshu Chubanshe] [Encyclopedia of China Publishing House].

Zhonggong Zhongyang Guowuyuan Yinfa [中共中央国务院印发)] [Chinese Communist Party Central Committee State Council Publication]. 1993. "中国教育改革和发展纲要 [Zhongguo Jiaoyu Gaige He Fazhan Gangyao] [Outline of China's Education Reforms and Development]." 人民日报 [Renmin Ribao] [People's Daily]. February 27.

Zhu, Chao [朱潮], ed. 1988. 中外医学教育史 [Zhong Wai Yixue Jiaoyu Shi] [History of Medical Education in China and Abroad]. Shanghai: 上海醫科大學出版社 [Shanghai Yike Daxue Chubanshe] [Shanghai Medical University Press].

Zhu, Chao [朱潮] and Weifeng Zhang [张慰丰]. 1990. 新中国医学教育史 [Xin Zhongguo Yixue Jiaoyu Shi] [History of Medical Education in New China]. Beijing: 北京医科大学: 中国协和医科大学 [Beijing Yike Daxue, Zhongguo Hexie Yike Daxue Lianhe Chubanshe] [Associated Press of Beijing Medical University and Peking Union Medical University].

4 Mission and Modernity: The History and Development of Medical Education in Taiwan

Ming-Jung Ho, Kevin Shaw, Julie Shih, and Yu-Ting Chiu

THIS CHAPTER WILL review the history of medical education in Taiwan, highlighting major external forces that have shaped its development and internal actors, factors, and institutions. Then proceeding to contemporary challenges and reforms, we will place the current state of Taiwanese medical education in historical and regional perspective.

Throughout Taiwan's history, the development of medical education has served as a vehicle for modernization. Whether negotiating the relationship between traditional Chinese medicine (TCM) and Western biomedicine, old and new political regimes, or local conditions and globalization, Taiwanese medical education has faced the task of continually synthesizing its many influences. On one level, the story of Taiwan's medical education can be told through the arrival and departure of foreign regimes. Yet, a history of medical education on the island would be incomplete without emphasizing the unique political agency of physicians and, more broadly, the role that Taiwanese people and institutions have played in making their medical education globally viable and locally coherent. A broad view of Taiwan's medical education in the past and present will foreground both the powerful international forces that have shaped its institutions and the agency of Taiwanese medical educators and students themselves.

A Summative History

Colonization of Taiwan by the Dutch and Spanish in the early seventeenth century first brought Western medicine to Taiwan (then called "Formosa"). Before then, indigenous practitioners included TCM practitioners, orthopedists, acupuncturists, herbalists, midwives, and folk medicine practitioners (Watt 2008). When the Qing Dynasty took control of the island in 1683, TCM became the dominant medical paradigm because of its popularity among the immigrants from mainland China, consisting of herbal and Han medicine based on theories of yin-yang and the five elements (H. Chiang 2007a). From 1865 to 1895, toward the end of Qing rule, medical missionaries seeded the development of modern medicine in Taiwan. From 1895–1945, Japanese colonization further contributed to the diffusion of Western medicine, including the development of Taiwan's modern medical education system and national public health reforms. With the advent of US aid, the Anglo-American system of medical education supplanted the German-Japanese system established under the Japanese, introducing clerkship programs and rigorous licensure standards that continue to distinguish the professional status of physicians in the Republic of China today.

Missionary Medicine

In the nineteenth century, modern medicine spread to Taiwan through colonialism and the work of medical missionaries. The Qing Dynasty suffered defeat in the Second Opium War (1856–1860), signing the Treaty of Tianjin 1858 and the Treaty of Peking 1860. These treaties opened the gates of mainland China and Taiwan to foreign missionaries and business owners, rendering trading ports key sites of outside influence.

Following the treaties, Great Britain set up agencies to take charge of medical work for the Chinese Imperial Maritime Customs Service. Dr. Patrick Manson, known at the time as the "father of tropical medicine," represented the customs medical officers responsible for implementing health safety measures across Pacific borders (S. Chen 2002). Dr. Manson was introduced to Taiwan by his colleague, Dr. James L. Maxwell, who moved to Taiwan in 1865 to preach and practice medicine, the first in a series of Presbyterian missionaries. Following after Dr. Maxwell, missionaries George L. Mackay and David Landsborough founded the first Western medical institutions in northern and central Taiwan (Yeh 2003; Chou et al. 2012). Between 1865 and 1895, missionaries established several institutions of Western medicine, including the Mackay Hospital in Taipei, the Gu Lau Hospital in Tainan, and the Christian Hospital in Changhua (Sun, Ho, and Chen 2013). Many local youth worked as assistants at missionary hospitals, learning Western medicine and eventually obtaining certificates to practice as independent physicians (Watt 2008). Local students received basic medical education at newly established institutions, planting the seeds of modern medicine in Taiwan (Yeh 2003).

Japanese Colonization

In 1895, China lost to Japan in the First Sino-Japanese War, and Taiwan was handed over as a concession. When Japanese troops occupied Taiwan, they discovered they were losing more soldiers to disease and poor sanitary conditions than to combat. Thus, Japan's colonial government (the Taiwan Government-General) prioritized the development of modern medicine (H. Chiang 2007b).

Following the Meiji Restoration in 1868, Japan had adopted German medical practices and ideology, which viewed wide-scale public health intervention as a duty of the state (M. Liu 1997). Based on the ideology of state medicine, the government established state-run centers of medical education and the first formal medical education curriculum (M. Liu 2009). More so than any other profession, the colonial government encouraged the Taiwanese to study medicine (C. Chiu, Arrigo, and Tsai 2009).

Goto Shimpei, a Japanese politician and physician trained in Germany, took charge of the island's civil administration and led the establishment of medical and public health infrastructure. His policies included implementing the tap-water and sewer system, malaria and plague prevention, opium regulation, and the establishment of public hospitals and associations such as the National Health Services (M. Liu 2004; Fan 2005; Juang 1998). In 1897, Goto's administration established the Native Doctor Training Institute at Taipei Hospital to train Taiwanese locals, which included those with family ties to mainland China, as well as indigenous people. (The institute was the historical nucleus of National Taiwan University College of Medicine.) In 1899, the institute became the Medical School of Taiwan Government-General and began enrolling students across the country in a five-year curriculum. At first, few locals applied, viewing medicine as an unfamiliar and low-grade occupation (Chou et al. 2012). After the implementation of entrance exams, the number of applicants gradually rose as medicine became associated with pride and status (Y. Fan 2005). As a result of Goto's policies, medicine gained professional status and prestige, becoming one of few professions that provided Taiwanese locals with upward mobility in a colonial system (Chou et al. 2012).

As part of the Japanese government's modernization project, medical education followed a pattern of continual expansion. With the passage of the Taiwan Education Law, the medical curriculum expanded to encompass four years of preparatory courses and four years of undergraduate courses, eight years altogether. The Medical School of Taiwan Government-General thus became the Taihoku Specialist Medical School, recruiting graduates of five-year middle schools as of 1922. In 1928, Taihoku Imperial University broke ground as the first university-level institution, and in 1936, it opened its Department of Medicine, which absorbed the Taihoku Specialist Medical School (Juang 1998). The new hybrid institution recruited graduates of three-year high schools, elevating physician training from the junior college to the university level.

During the Japanese colonial regime, medicine was institutionalized as "a tool both for civilizing the colonial subjects and for legitimizing the colonial regime" (M. Lo 2002, 52). Under this system, a class of Taiwanese physicians emerged that embodied ethnic professionalism: the fusion of medical professionalism and deference to Japanese superiors with a mixed sense of ethnic and national identity.

The "in-betweenness" of Taiwanese doctors ideally situated them to carry out the public health care projects of the Japanese state in areas where locals mistrusted Japanese officials (ibid.). Over time, the state granted greater organizational autonomy to Taiwanese physicians, who were able to carve out a space for anticolonial resistance (ibid.), even as they benefited from their profession's high level of integration into the colonial system (ibid.). These "national physicians" and "ethnic professionals" contested discrimination as it existed in professional practice and medical education (ibid.). Although locked within a professional pyramid that rendered them subordinate to Japanese physicians, Taiwanese doctors enjoyed a favorable market outlook and expanding educational opportunities. Simultaneously subordinated by the colonial state and distanced from the public by their class privilege, Taiwanese physicians developed a hybrid identity that must be understood in order to comprehend the fusion of national mission and modernity that characterized early medical education in Taiwan and that would influence its development under the Kuomintang (KMT).

Over the first four decades of the twentieth century, traditional Chinese medicine gradually declined in prominence as biomedicine became the dominant mode of care and treatment on the island. In 1901, the Japanese government passed regulations mandating that all practitioners of TCM register with police authorities or else forfeit their right to practice. These regulations effectively instituted a bottleneck for the entry of Chinese-herbal doctors to the field, as schools of biomedicine became the only legitimate sites of medical instruction (Yao 2003). The year 1920 marks the watershed point at which doctors trained in biomedicine outnumbered TCM practitioners for the first time in Taiwanese history (*Taiwan Sheng Xingzheng Zhangguan Gongshu Tongjishi* 1946). The Japanese government continued to hold licensing examinations for traditional practitioners until the 1930s, by which time the number of Chinese-herbal practitioners had declined significantly. (The decline of TCM under Japanese governance is discussed further in Kenichi Ohmi's chapter in this volume.) Meanwhile, the Japanese government authorized the creation of private medical schools in Taiwan. The combination of these two policies, in the long term, led to the gradual increase of physicians trained in Western scientific medicine and the decrease of practitioners of Chinese medicine. In the short term, however, the decline of traditional medicine had a drastic effect on Taiwan's medical workforce. Between 1906 and 1940, the Taiwanese ratio of doctors to population decreased at an annualized rate of 0.8 percent. The increase in Japanese-trained physicians was simply too small to make up for the gap left by traditional medicine (M. Liu 2009).

At the time of Japan's forfeiture of Taiwan in 1945, Taiwanese medical education had seen fifty years of change under colonization. With the rise of medical schools and a formalized curriculum, medicine gained respect as a profession.

Taiwanese medical students often shared a close pupil-teacher relationship with their foreign instructors (ibid.), developing strong bonds with their Japanese mentors while maintaining antipathy for the colonial government (Chou et al. 2012). While medicine gained professional status under the Japanese, comparable educational standards were not implemented for other health professions. As a result, nurses and midwives were trained and supervised by physicians, rather than practicing independently of physicians. Additionally, the state stripped the field of pharmacy of its professional status, leaving only physicians with the ability to legally prescribe medications. The colonial government suppressed the development of Chinese medicine, and Western scientific medicine became the mainstream (M. Liu 2004). As the Japanese government withdrew from Taiwan, it left behind a legacy marked by significant growth in medical education but also by inter-professional disparity.

The Republic of China

In August 1945, Japanese colonization of Taiwan officially ended. In October, the government of the Republic of China established itself in Taiwan, causing shifts in the island's disease burden and its systems of medical education, including a change in the primary language of instruction from Japanese to Mandarin Chinese. During the initial stage of Taiwan's transfer from Japanese colonial authority to the Republic of China, diseases resurfaced that had once been brought under control, including malaria, smallpox, and cholera. Epidemic prevention and physician training thus became urgent matters of course, while political instability triggered a crisis in the licensure and supply of qualified physicians. Concurrently, an expansion in the presence of the United States led to an influx of resources for medical education, as well as changes in medical institutions, curricula, and values.

At the outset, the transition of the KMT government to Taiwan had deleterious effects on the training and licensure of physicians. In the absence of a stable regulatory authority, licensing regulations for new physicians loosened (T. Chiang 1995). At the time, most practicing doctors had received their training during Japanese rule. KMT officials in charge of issuing medical licenses often abused their power, licensing illegal and untrained doctors and questionably trained military doctors who accompanied the government's exodus from the mainland. In 1950, the Taiwanese Doctors' Association pressed the government to revise the Physician Act and enforce a more rigorous system of licensure. On May 26, 1967, the Legislative Yuan signed the Physician Act amendment into law. The next year, the Examination Yuan, a separate branch of government in charge of holding national examinations, determined that all applicants wishing to receive a physician's license must be checked for proper certification and pass a screening interview. Although the law took seventeen years to pass, the government's strict ban on fake and unlicensed doctors reasserted the importance of legitimate and regulated medical education (T. Chiang 1995).

US Aid and Influence

Following the relocation of the Kuomintang in 1949 and the outbreak of the Korean War in 1950, the United States sought to intensify its geopolitical presence in East Asia. Accordingly, it initiated a fifteen-year period of aid to Taiwan (Y. Fan 1999), triggering a shift in the dominant paradigm of medical education from the German-Japanese to the American model (Yeh 2004). In 1953, the Mutual Security Agency's (MSA) Mission to China sent a delegation of US medical and pharmaceutical experts to evaluate Taiwan's health needs. They found that wartime damage and neglect had left medical facilities and infrastructure at National Taiwan University (NTU, formerly Taihoku Imperial University) in poor condition (Watt 2008). During the war, American bombers had mistaken the NTU School of Medicine for a factory, and the destroyed areas had not yet been rebuilt (Humphreys 2008). The delegation sent detailed recommendations to the US Department of State to assist in the medical school's recovery and reconstruction. Thereafter, the MSA made NTU a focal point of its health aid plan (T. Yang 2008).

After the war, international exchanges brought American leadership and forms of health care to Taiwan, establishing strong ties between American and Taiwanese institutions of medical education. Wilbert C. Davison, PhD, from Duke University helped import the clerkship system to Taiwan's clinical education system (Hsieh 2004), and in 1954, the United States sponsored the president and vice president of NTU School of Medicine for a period of study at Duke University. Upon their return, they set about revising basic medical courses, dividing each specialty into different subspecialties, and separating fifth- and sixth-year students for small group instruction. This trend of international exchange included students themselves: in 1955, a Taiwanese student cohort embarked for study in America (T. Yang 2008).

At the governmental level, the KMT received financial support from both the US government and the China Medical Board (CMB), an independent American foundation. CMB funded new facilities and faculty training at NTU College of Medicine (including the School of Medicine, School of Nursing, and School of Pharmacy) (Xiong, Chiang, and Cheng 1990), the creation of a library system at Kaohsiung Medical University containing medical and other literature (C. Liu 2013), and the creation of new medical schools in Taiwan, including Taipei Medical University and the National Defense Medical Center (NDMC) (Sytwu 2013). The relationships between NDMC, CMB, and the American Bureau for Medical Aid to China (ABMAC) established lasting channels of communication between Taiwan and international actors (D. Tsai 2009).

Two Leading Medical Education Institutions

After the KMT established itself on the island, two of Taiwan's most important medical education institutions came into prominence. First, the Faculty of Medicine at Taihoku Imperial University became the National Taiwan University College of Medicine (NTUCM) in 1945. At the time, the medical school curriculum was a five-year program for high school graduates. By 1948, the curriculum for the fulfillment of a bachelor of medicine degree had grown to seven years: two years of preparatory courses, four years of undergraduate medical courses, and one year of internship. Under the new government, NTUCM switched from the German-style workshop system established under the Japanese to the American-style credit system.

Second, the National Defense Medical Center (NDMC) relocated from the mainland to Taiwan, taking on a leading role in medical education. NDMC was established by graduates of Peking Union Medical College (PUMC) in China to support the nationalist army, first against the Japanese and then during the Chinese Civil War (Watt 2008). When the Nationalists and NDMC collectively retreated to Taiwan, they brought with them PUMC's residency training system, inherited from the United States, as well as much of PUMC's former curriculum and leadership. The new residency training system stimulated changes in medical training at NTUCM as well as Taiwan more broadly. NDMC became the center for professional nursing education on the island. Headed by General Chow Mei-yu, a PUMC graduate and ardent nationalist, NDMC's nursing program benefited from the pro-America, anti-Japanese scrutiny of health policymakers (T. Lo 2008). During the early stages of transition, NDMC proposed a merger with NTUCM. Although this did not come to fruition, NDMC brought experienced medical educators and American-style training to Taiwan, challenging NTUCM's national dominance in the medical arena (D. Tsai 2009).

The Rise, Fall, and Rise of Private Medical Schools

In the latter half of the twentieth century, strong interest in medical education among young people, especially the children of physicians, led to the creation of private medical schools, versions of which had been established under Japanese colonization (T. Chiang 1995). In 1954, Dr. Tu Tsung-ming left his post as dean of NTUCM, where he had pioneered diagnostics and therapeutic treatment for opium addiction, to establish Kaohsiung Medical College, the first private medical school in Taiwan. From the 1950s to the 1970s, private institutions were established across the island, including China Medical College, Taipei Medical College, and Chung Shan Medical and Dental College (Hsieh 2004). Although the establishment of private medical schools increased the overall number of medical schools, and therefore the number of health professionals who graduated each year, additional schools could not solve fundamental shortage issues, which stemmed from large numbers of physicians retiring.

In 1972, the government froze the growth of private institutions of higher education, citing concerns with the quality of existing private schools, which were still in a nascent state of development (P. Lin 2006; C. Yang 2007; H. Liu 2011; Wang 1996). This policy necessitated the establishment of more public schools of medicine, including Yang Ming School of Medicine in 1975 and National Cheng Kung University School of Medicine in 1983. Yang Ming School of Medicine, in particular, facilitated the training of nationally sponsored physicians, who received educational funding in exchange for six years of public health and medical service in places lacking medical resources and personnel (Y. Chen 1997). The government also mandated that each medical school increase its number of admitted students, subsidizing their tuition. In addition to the traditional seven-year medical program, schools began piloting a five-year program for postgraduate entry in 1982 (T. Chiang 1995).

The government allowed the establishment of private medical schools to resume in 1985. Most funding for private schools originated from business or religious groups (P. Lin 2006). The first business-managed hospital, Chang Gung Hospital, was established by Formosa Plastic Group, which also funded the creation of the Chang Gung School of Medicine in 1987 (Editorial Board of *Medicine Today* 1987). In the 1990s, private medical institutions were begun under the religious aegis of both Buddhism and Catholicism (Fu Jen Catholic University College of Medicine; Tzu Chi University College of Medicine). In 2013, I-shou University received permission to establish a medical school with funding from the E United Group, offering four-year postgraduate degrees with English lectures (I-Shou University College of Medicine. This most recent addition to Taiwan's medical education landscape reflects the ongoing internationalization of higher education.

Quality Assurance

As American aid gradually withdrew, full authority over medical education policy returned to the government, and the Department of Health was established in 1971. To ensure that medical personnel maintained their skills, the Department of Health (DOH) established continuing education systems for fourteen types of medical personnel, making participation in continuing education courses a precondition for the renewal of licenses every six years. The 1985 amendment of the Physician Act established separate licensure pathways for physicians in specialty professions.

In 1998, a review from the US National Committee on Foreign Medical Education and Accreditation (NCFMEA) found Taiwan's medical education "noncomparable" to that of the United States, noting that the country lacked a dedicated system of accreditation for medical education. The Ministry of Education and Taiwan's medical educators responded by enlisting the nonprofit National Health Research Institute to develop a medical accreditation system. In 1999, the Taiwan Medical Accreditation Council (TMAC) was established with funding from the Department of Health and was found "comparable" by the NCFMEA, which reviews accreditation bodies (Chou et al. 2012). The TMAC standards were reviewed and revised in 2013.

In 2003, Severe Acute Respiratory Syndrome (SARS) struck Taiwan (Centers for Disease Control, Republic of China [Taiwan] 2013). The SARS outbreak revealed that many physicians were deficient in the competencies needed to care for patients with illnesses falling outside their specialty or subspecialty. In August 2003, the Department of Health launched a three-month "Postgraduate General Medical Training" (PGMT) program with a focus on providing general medical education, which they extended to one year in August 2006 (Hsieh 2003). At present, all medical graduates are required to take the PGMT course before taking the specialty board examinations (Y. Chen et al. 2013).

Traditional Medicine

Traditional Chinese medicine was eventually restored to public practice during the postwar period. Lacking a system for licensure or standardization, however, traditional medicine's resurgence contributed to the disarray and deregulation of the medical professions at large. In 2000, the licensure system for Chinese medicine went through an overhaul, requiring traditional practitioners to undergo coursework in anatomy and physiology alongside classical Chinese medicine (Chiu, Arrigo, and Tsai 2009). Today, four programs of Chinese medicine exist in Taiwan. Although students of traditional medicine are required to undergo Western basic science and clinical curricula, they must choose whether to pursue licensure for traditional medicine or biomedicine, as one cannot hold both licenses simultaneously.

National Health Insurance

Physicians played a significant role in the democratization movement that gripped Taiwan in the 1980s and 1990s. Their political activism fueled demands for equitable, universal health insurance. Though strapped by financial difficulties, the government faced overwhelming political pressure to implement comprehensive health coverage. The Council for Economic Planning and Development started planning a social welfare system in 1984, calling for the implementation of National Health Insurance by the year 2000. Beginning in 1986, a chain of political developments unfolded: the declaration of martial law, the passage of the Civil Organizations Act, and the reelection of the congress. Under pressure of legislative elections in 1995 and an impending presidential election in March 1996, the government accelerated voting on health insurance. National Health Insurance (NHI) was hastily implemented on March 1, 1995 (T. Chiang 2003). Since then, the government has performed the role of planner, policymaker, price-setter, payer, and consumer representative in the health care system.

Under NHI, coverage is compulsory for all citizens and includes a comprehensive benefits package. NHI is funded primarily through a payroll tax, and each visit requires a copayment in order to share costs and reduce unnecessary usage. Nonetheless, NHI's implementation initially resulted in a boom in service volume. In 2004, NHI reformed its finances according to the global budget system approach, effectively controlling the growth of medical expenditures while increasing the financial burden borne by patients. The NHI global budget system has both positive and negative implications for medical professionalism. While it addresses the incentives that previously led to a large increase in service quantity and density, the pressure placed on hospitals to control costs has shifted the burden of paying for many pharmaceuticals onto patients and resulted in patients being prematurely discharged or repeatedly transferred. Moreover, it raises the incentives for doctors to shift costs onto patients by, for instance, suggesting patients undertake high-tech diagnostics at their own expense. Overall, while more sustainable from a financial perspective, the new system raises concerns of ill effects for doctor-patient relationships and overall service quality (J. Chiu 2015), posing continuing challenges for medical professionalism.

NHI reimburses clinical instructors for patient care but not for instruction, and this likely minimizes their uncompensated teaching time. Only a minority of physicians at teaching hospitals have faculty appointments at medical schools, and thus a secondary source of income from teaching. Conversely, most teaching hospital staff receive compensation solely for clinical services and lack a significant financial incentive to focus on teaching (Humphreys 2008).

A Summary of Internal Factors and Actors

A history of medical education in Taiwan would not be complete without an account of the local factors, individuals, and institutions that shaped its development. Medical education institutions established under the Japanese and continued under the KMT shaped medical professionals with a strong sense of national mission. Historical shifts in governance triggered major changes in medical educational culture, institutions, and practice. With the KMT's relocation to Taiwan came a surge of immigration, bringing new epidemiological threats and populations to be serviced. The KMT also brought NDMC with it, changing the institutional landscape of medicine. In the late twentieth

94 | *Medical Education in East Asia*

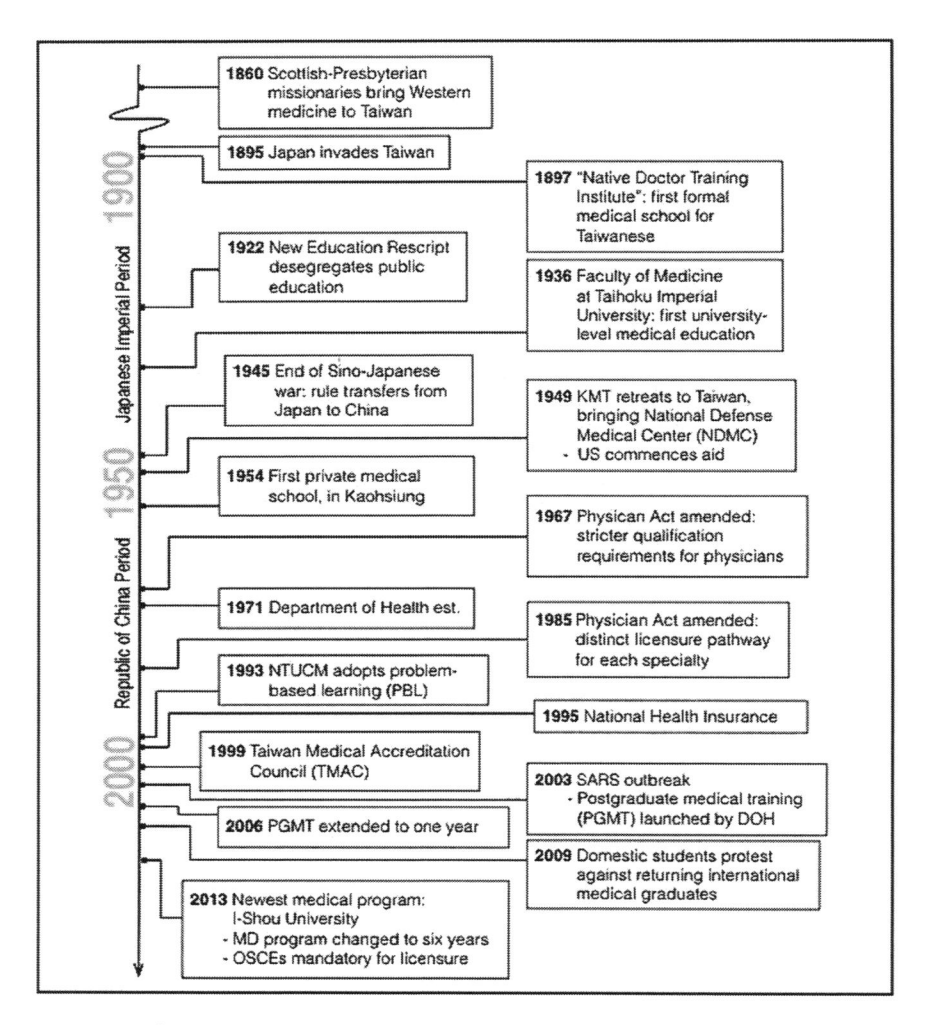

Fig. 4.1. Timeline: Medical Education in Taiwan.

century, Taiwan's economic transformation shifted the disease burden toward noncommunicable diseases, making physician training a priority of the state. In the face of these pressures, medical educators and policymakers targeted underfunded medical education and corrupt, inadequate licensure systems for reform. Recently, reforms in Taiwan have also sought to integrate humanism more deeply into curriculums in response to a global push by medical educators to promote professionalism. Medical professionalism entails behaviors such as respecting patients and communicating effectively with them. These competencies were not emphasized in Taiwan's traditional, lecture-based model of medical education, where students entered medicine directly from high school without exposure to the humanities. Today, admission to medical school is regulated partly by an examination system grounded in academic meritocracy, though increasingly, schools are allowing for entry via personal application and high school recommendation. Set in the context of globalization and increasingly frequent international exchanges, medical education in Taiwan continues to develop and change.

Current Landscape

In Taiwan, medical schools offer seven-year programs with undergraduate entry. In 2013, medical school programs were changed to six years followed by a postgraduate internship, though students enrolled prior to 2013 will follow the seven-year program to its completion. Only one school currently operates a dual-entry system with an additional four-year graduate-entry program. The following section summarizes the current state of medical education for physicians, including institutional and instructional design (student selection process, curriculums, teaching hospitals, faculty development, postgraduate training, accreditation, and licensure systems), followed by a brief overview of nursing and public health education. It then zooms out to look at developments in medical education from a systems-level perspective, addressing challenges such as cultivating students' clinical competency, developing high-quality teaching faculty, and integrating social sciences and the humanities into medical education.

Today, Taiwanese medical schools accept a total of 1,300 students, an annual enrollment capped by the Ministry of Health. Enrollment for other types of medical personnel is also subject to the quota system. Applications must be submitted to and reviewed by the Ministry of Education prior to the establishment of training programs (Ministry of Health and Welfare 2013).

Given Taiwan's population of approximately 23 million, there are fifteen physicians per 10,000 people, lower than the average for OECD (Organization for Economic Cooperation and Development) countries. Between 1982 and 1991, five medical schools attempted a postbaccalaureate, dual-enrollment system, but currently only one continues the practice.

Selection of Medical Students

Upon graduation from high school, medical students in Taiwan are selected using three criteria: the National College Entrance Exam, personal applications, and high school recommendations. Previously, medical schools relied exclusively on national exam scores to assess prospective students, a method that fell under heavy criticism by the American NCFMEA in 1988 for lacking consideration of personal characteristics. Increasingly, Taiwanese medical schools have adopted a mixed-methods approach to medical school admissions. Today, 40 percent of enrollment is determined through an application process that includes academic records and personal interviews (Chou et al. 2012).

Medical School Curriculums

In 1992, Taiwanese medical education began a process of broad-based reforms. Among other goals, the reforms emphasized: self-directed and active learning; the integration of an interdisciplinary science curriculum; earlier clinical exposure to enhance clinical skills acquisition; and better integration of the humanities, social sciences, and liberal arts into premed curriculums (Tsou et al. 2009). Taiwan's medical curriculum is divided into premedical education for the first two years, basic sciences in the following two years, and clinical medicine in the final three years, for the seven-year program (for students who entered before 2013), or two years of clinical medicine for the new six-year program (effective for students entering after 2013).

Curricular reforms in Taiwan have sought to promote self-directed learning through the incorporation of problem-based learning (PBL) curriculums, beginning with National Taiwan University College of Medicine in 1993. PBL emphasizes experiential learning through problem cases, implemented in small groups led by tutors, in contrast to pedagogies focusing on rote memorization. Pioneered by McMaster University in the late 1960s (Lee and Kwan 1997), PBL has since seen rapid uptake by medical schools around the world, exemplifying the global diffusion of Anglo-Saxon teaching models to developing country contexts (Stevens and Goulbourne 2012). PBL supports a variety of learning activities, such as lectures, laboratory exercises, and clinical skills teaching. Tools used to evaluate student learning include oral feedback, written feedback, and a summative assessment scored in part by the tutor. As an example, Fu Jen Medical School launched a PBL curriculum for its third- and fourth-year students, with three-hour sessions three times a week in the third year and twice a week in the fourth year. In these case-based tutorial sessions, students are placed into small groups of six to eight with a tutor to guide them through the activities (Tsou et al. 2009).

Potential benefits of a PBL curriculum include improvements to students' clinical reasoning processes, self-directed learning skills, and ability to apply scientific knowledge to clinical cases. Successfully implementing PBL, however, requires close attention to the cultural and social conditions that underlie effective teamwork, especially in medical schools that have a diverse and heterogeneous student population (Stevens and Goulbourne 2012). In the Fu Jen study, students cited shortcomings in the depth and completeness of the PBL curriculum, saying they did not feel confident handling diseases not covered by their PBL cases (Tsou et al. 2009). An evaluation of the PBL curriculum at Kaohsiung Medical University, meanwhile, found issues with tutor training and staffing, leading to organizational reforms (Y. Lin et al. 2009). Since 2002, all eleven medical schools in Taiwan have implemented the PBL curriculum in combination with other programs.

Teaching Hospitals

Teaching hospitals are accredited facilities for training future physicians and other health care professionals. In Taiwan, teaching hospitals are classified into two levels: A-level hospitals are larger and offer tertiary care, while B-level hospitals are smaller community institutions. Set standards require both types of hospitals to have an adequate number of qualified teaching physicians and teaching resources. The standards stipulate basic requirements for hours of bedside teaching, number of publications, and training, teaching, and research expenses (Huang, Wung, and Yang 2009). In 2011, the DOH has revised the Teaching Hospital Accreditation Standards to expand accreditation of teaching hospitals to fourteen different categories of medical personnel (Ministry of Health and Welfare 2013). Medical schools are affiliated with teaching hospitals where students receive clinical training. Hospitals affiliated with medical schools must be DOH-accredited teaching hospitals. However, not all DOH-accredited teaching hospitals are affiliated with medical schools.

Faculty Development

Both government and professional bodies have worked to improve medical education at the instructor, resident, and student levels. In 2006, the Taiwan Association of Medical Education (TAME) assisted teaching hospitals in the establishment of General Medical Training Demonstration Centers to promote training for clinical instructors and graduates in general medicine. Clinical instructors are trained to educate postgraduate residents in the core competencies of the Accreditation Council for Graduate Medical Education (ACGME) (Accreditation Council for Graduate Medical Education; F. Lee et al. 2011). Instructors of allied health professionals have to meet DOH qualification regulations of teaching hospitals as well (Ministry of Health and Welfare 2014).

Supervising Bodies for Medical Accreditation

A spectrum of national supervisory organizations has evolved for accreditation, including the Ministry of Education (MOE), Taiwan Medical Accreditation Council (TMAC), and Ministry of Health and Welfare (former Department of Health). These organizations also issue recommendations for reform. The MOE used separate accreditation systems for various medical institutions until TMAC was established in 1999 as an independent organization for medical education accreditation, modeled after the Liaison Committee on Medical Education

(LCME) of the United States and the Australian Medical Council (Lai 2009). TMAC's accreditation standards were recently revised with a focus on enforceability, and new standards have been implemented as of autumn 2014. The Ministry of Health and Welfare is in charge of the regulation of teaching hospitals and health care professionals.

Licensure Exam

Since its introduction in the 1990s, the Objective Structured Clinical Examination (OSCE) has grown in importance as a formative assessment in Taiwan. Starting in 2013, following two large-scale pilots conducted in 2011 and 2012 (C. Lin et al. 2013) passing the OSCE is required for Taiwanese medical students taking the licensure exam to practice medicine. 2013 saw 1,263 final-year medical students in Taiwan enroll in the national OSCE. Those who fail the exam are not qualified to take the medical licensure examination administered by the Ministry of Examination (Dong 2013).

Postgraduate Training

The Postgraduate General Medical Training Program has been promoted by the DOH with the goal of improving physician competencies in primary and holistic care. Originally begun as a three-month postgraduate general medical training program, its second phase began in 2006 and extended the training period to six months. Having entered a third phase in July 2011, the program now offers a full year of postgraduate training (Ministry of Health and Welfare 2013). Today, all medical graduates must complete a full year of postgraduate training program approved by the Ministry of Education and demonstrate competencies in general medicine before they can enter a specialty residency program.

Nursing Education

Currently, there are a total of forty institutions offering basic nursing education, producing 14,000 graduates per year (L. Chao 2012). There are thirteen institutions under the Ministry of Education's Higher Education Division and two under the Ministry of Education's Technical and Vocational Education Department. In addition, there is one department of nursing at the National Defense Medical Center of the Ministry of National Defense. There are two types of curriculum in vocational academic schools: a two-year junior college system and a five-year junior college system. Some universities and technical schools offer two-year technical programs, four-year technical programs, or four-year undergraduate programs, resulting in a total of five different curriculums for nursing education in Taiwan. Two degrees are offered to graduates, the associate degree in nursing (ADN) and the bachelor of science in nursing (BSN). Diverse student backgrounds and different maturity levels have presented a significant challenge to nursing schools, impacting the quality and effectiveness of education, making it difficult to maintain a set standard (Yu, Dai, and Yeh 2010). To improve the quality of nursing education, the Ministry of Education established the Taiwan Nursing Accreditation Council (TNAC) in 2006 to oversee nursing program evaluation (Higher Education Evaluation and Accredication Council of Taiwan 2013).

Public Health Education

Taiwan established its public health education system during the initial stages of transfer to rule by the Republic of China. There are currently fifty-four undergraduate programs (up from fourteen programs in the 1980s) and thirty-four graduate programs for public health, including general colleges and universities and technical and vocational schools. Although no new departments of public health have been established since the 1990s, the number of health care administration programs has increased from four to twenty-seven since the year 2000. Environmental and occupational health programs, as well as other related health departments, have also seen growth. Around 5,000 students graduate from public health programs annually. Until recently, due to differences in teaching faculty and course focus among various programs, little national uniformity existed with regard to standardized course requirements or core competencies. In 2009, the Taiwan Public Health Association implemented a training program, modeled after the Basic Level in Public Health Core Competency Examination (BPHCE) used in the United States, in order to encourage competition and improve the quality of public health education (W. Chen and T. Chiang 2010).

Current and Future Challenges

Clinical competencies, graduating students' suitability to practice medicine, the need for high-quality teaching faculty, and a changing landscape for physician licensing all pose challenges to medical education and the practice of medicine in Taiwan.

Firstly, cultivating clinical competence in Taiwanese medical students is a major area of concern. A 2012 survey found that only 70 percent expressed satisfaction with their medical education, but even fewer—56 percent—expressed confidence in their primary care skills (W. Chan et al. 2012). Although students may demonstrate knowledge of clinical procedures in a classroom setting, they encounter challenges putting that knowledge into practice in a clinical environment. Medical students in Taiwan rely too much on class notes and past exam papers because their assessments are largely based on written examinations rather than other methods of performance evaluation (W. Chan 2013). Clinical competence could be improved through earlier exposure to patients, reducing classroom-based instruction during the undergraduate years, increasing postgraduate training in clinical skills, and more rigorous evaluation of clinical competence.

Other factors beyond clinical skills may call into question students' suitability to practice medicine upon graduation. An underlying problem is the heavy emphasis that Taiwanese schools have historically placed on national exam scores during the admissions process, although interviews are growing in importance as a method for screening out unsuitable personalities (W. Chan 2013). In addition, medical schools lack an effective exit mechanism for students once they matriculate. If a student finds medicine unsuitable and wishes to pursue a different field of study, she or he would have to start another degree program from the beginning. This inflexible system discourages students from changing professions, likely funneling students into the profession who might be better suited elsewhere. When dissatisfied students lack an established pathway for switching out of medicine, it may affect their professionalism upon entering practice.

More good teachers are also needed. Due to an overemphasis on research in the selection and promotion of faculty (W. Chan 2013) and the fact that NHI does not compensate faculty physicians for teaching, not many physicians are attracted to teaching (Chu, Weed, and Yang 2009). Furthermore, clinical educators lack a teaching-friendly clinical environment and are pressured by NHI's system to devote more time to patient care and less time to teaching.

The turbulent politics of international medical education have led to recent changes for Taiwanese who decide to study abroad for their medical degrees. In 2002, the government lowered barriers to reentry for degree-holders from specific "developed" regions, a category that came to encompass Poland once it joined the EU in 2004. Taiwanese students obtaining medical degrees in Poland became the focus of a public controversy, feeding skepticism toward the academic and clinical capabilities of returning international medical graduates (IMGs). Poland's medical programs offered English-language programs targeting international students, with curriculums structured around US standards (Hodges et al. 2009). As more Taiwanese IMGs returned to practice with Polish degrees, domestic students took note and protested, both online and in the streets. Claims of unfairness dominated the exchange on both sides. Domestic students targeted the rigor and legitimacy of Polish programs, complaining that they lacked internships and were shorter in duration, although discussion of the latter point sometimes obscured the distinction between Poland's four-year postgraduate and six-year undergraduate degrees. Moreover, they emphasized that Polish international medical programs operated on a for-profit basis and admitted students on the basis of applications rather than examinations, without the pressure of an enrollment cap and with higher tuition rates than Taiwan. In turn, graduates of Polish schools defended the rigor and technical strength of their education, noting a lower student retention rate among Polish schools than among Taiwanese schools and arguing for equal opportunity to participate in the medical marketplace (Ho et al. 2015). The movement to increase screening procedures for returning IMGs attracted attention and support from DOH officials and from others active in the government, media, and public. Outnumbered and isolated, the overseas medical students faced an uphill political battle, not least against an atmosphere of stigma, exemplified by attempts by some citizens to track the whereabouts of practitioners with Polish medical degrees through online lists and even a mobile phone application. As of March 2014, a one-year domestic internship had gone into effect for all IMGs seeking licensure, while the degree-qualification exam remained stalled in the Legislative Yuan.

In addition to concerns about quality and fitness to practice medicine after graduation either in Taiwan or internationally, Taiwan currently also faces health systems challenges, such as recruiting personnel in internal medicine, surgery, OB-GYN, and pediatrics due to low reimbursement for primary care by the National Health Insurance rates and lifestyle preferences of the young physicians (Cheng 2013). Other factors making primary care specialties less attractive include increasing lawsuits for malpractice and emergency room violence, such as reported cases of physical assault on doctors in response to long ER waiting times (Chang 2012).

Current Reforms and Developments

In March 2009, a working group composed of deans and presidents of various medical schools reached a consensus to reorganize the MD program, resulting in a change from seven to six years of instruction, followed by two years of postgraduate general medical training. Medical schools implemented this change in 2013, arguably the most important innovation in Taiwanese medical education within the last fifty years. These reforms have emphasized the importance of general medicine and the integration of basic sciences, social sciences, and the humanities with clinical medicine.

In response to the challenges posed in cutting costs and other structural factors, including rising costs for patients that complicate relationships with care providers, Taiwanese medical educators have led a reform movement for medical professionalism (Chou et al. 2012). Efforts have focused on integrating humanism into medical curriculums longitudinally, with additional postgraduate training. Schools have redesigned their curriculums to reinforce the lesson that "the essence of medicine should be social trust" (Chiu, Arrigo, and Tsai 2009, 513) and reaffirm the moral obligation of physicians toward their communities. They have done so partly through implementing educational strategies to develop students' competencies that meet local societal expectations (D. Tsai 2008), such as involving family members in medical decision-making. With regard to the admissions process, medical school officials are increasingly turning to admission interviews to screen for personal characteristics, balancing out the traditional overemphasis on academic and test performance (W. Chan 2013).

International migration has led to the emergence of an overseas community of Taiwanese-American medical educators that can serve as a powerful force for reform. Since the 1970s, the medical community in Taiwan has maintained close ties with the expatriate medical community in the United States. The mediating role of Taiwanese-American educators is especially important in light of the high overall respect held for US medical education, exemplified by the Ministry of Education's recommendations that the premedical curriculum be modeled on that of the United States (Chou et al. 2012). Since the 1990s, a significant number of Taiwanese-American doctors have returned, infusing Taiwanese universities with transnational training and expertise (Chiu, Arrigo, and Tsai 2009).

Past, Present, and Future Prospects

On one level, the story of Taiwan's medical education can be told with reference to foreign regimes of influence. Medical education in Taiwan is marked by the lasting influences of Japanese colonialism and US aid, which ushered in Western models of health care and training. Missionaries established the first modern medical institutions in Taiwan and the Japanese colonial government instituted widespread public health reforms and medical education based on German practices. Under colonial rule, physicians enjoyed an expansion of professional autonomy, relating in this context to self-regulation of the profession, as exemplified by licensure and the evolution of medical education to university status. Following the Korean War, US aid helped fund the growth of medical curriculums and the first residency and clerkship programs. US-Taiwan relations led to the replacement of German-Japanese modes of medical education with Anglo-American practices.

Inseparable from Taiwan's history of external forces influencing medical education are local persons, factors, and institutions. Since the formal development of modern biomedicine under the Japanese, professional autonomy, prestige, and a sense of public mission have served as hallmarks of the medical profession in Taiwan. Medical educators, in turn, have used their professional autonomy to push for change and reform. Taiwanese medical education exemplifies "hybridity." Whether at the individual level of physicians operating under colonial regimes or at the institutional level of curriculums imported from other countries, the "in-betweenness" of Taiwan and its people has served as a primary impetus for the growth of its medical institutions. Western medicine arrived on the island through foreign parties bearing the banner of modernization; today, Taiwanese educators and students continue to invoke modernization in the movement to better integrate medical humanities into professional education, countering concerns that students entering medical school out of high school may lack adequate exposure to the liberal arts and humanities.

While earlier stages of medical education focused on the cultivation of doctors *within* national borders, medical students are now studying across and beyond borders. The growing global character of Taiwanese medical education is reflected by the returning tide of Taiwanese physicians with degrees from other countries, in particular Poland and the United States. Eliciting sharply differing reactions from the Taiwanese medical establishment, both groups have nonetheless provoked dialogue and change. The return of Polish international medical graduates and the subsequent controversy have catalyzed tighter regulations on IMGs of all national stripes, including those who have studied in countries traditionally lionized as more developed. Meanwhile, returning Taiwanese-American physicians with years of US teaching experience have stimulated dialogue around curricular reform. In both cases, international exchanges have produced a force for change in Taiwanese medical education.

Going forward, Taiwanese medical education faces the twin challenges of maintaining competitiveness with global standards and addressing local needs. Thus, future reforms must be discussed in both their international and local contexts. The creation and evolution of the Taiwan Medical Accreditation Council, for instance, bears a close relationship with the movement to establish a reference standard for global accreditation of medical schools, which is led in part by the US Educational Commission for Foreign Medical Graduates (ECFMG). Given that ECFMG certification determines the eligibility of international medical graduates to enter medical training and practice in the United States—a popular destination for international medical graduates—countries may feel pressured to mold their accreditation standards after those used in the United States. When TMAC set about revising its standards in 2009, it sought to balance adherence to global standards while ensuring fit with local context. It did so through an iterative, collaborative process involving both international advisors and local stakeholders.

One suggestion is for the Department of Health to subsidize the cost of clinical teaching. Medical graduates lack confidence in their own clinical skills (W. Chan et al. 2012), signaling the need for greater attention to clinical teaching within curriculums. In cultivating the next generation of doctors, medical schools must prioritize humanism and altruism as fundamental attributes of a physician. In order to achieve the goal of health for all, Taiwan needs more primary care providers who are confident in their clinical skills and grounded in the principles of medical professionalism, as well as specialists within internal medicine, surgery, OB-GYN, and pediatrics.

Shared Challenges in Greater China

Although China, Hong Kong, and Taiwan have followed different paths in the development of medical education, they share a set of common challenges and approaches. First, teaching methods that encourage active learning, such as problem-based learning and team-based learning, have been implemented to counterbalance the teacher-centeredness of traditional Chinese education. In a move away from the lecture-intensive methods of traditional instruction, PBL curriculums implemented in Taiwan (Tsou et al. 2009) and Hong Kong (Tang 2001) have demonstrated promising student outcomes. In China, recent surveys have shown that, although the majority of sampled schools use PBL, there is only limited integration into the curriculums, due in part to the substantial investment of financial and faculty resources required (Fan et al. 2014).

Second, in terms of curricular structure, efforts are underway to counteract the fragmentation of academic disciplines by integrating basic sciences, the humanities, and social sciences with clinical medicine in Taiwan (Tsai et al. 2012), Hong Kong (Chan et al. 2011), and China (Hu et al. 2014). These efforts seek to balance a curriculum that is traditionally weighed toward the core sciences because students enter medical school as undergraduates selected through a test-based admissions process.

Third, regarding educational outcomes, competency-based medical education is being promoted through curricular reforms with the goal of equipping graduates not only with scientific knowledge, but also with the clinical competence necessary to deliver patient care as expected by society. New methods to evaluate clinical competence, such as the Objective Structured Clinical Examination (OSCE), are being developed and piloted. As of 2013, passing the national OSCE is required for medical licensure examination in Taiwan.

Fourth, the standardization of medical schools by a national accreditation system is under development in China, already implemented in Hong Kong, and recently reformed in Taiwan. The Taiwan Medical Accreditation Council has sought to revise the accreditation standards for medical education in Taiwan in a manner that both responds to local context and meets global standards, taking into account the structural, regulatory, and historical differences between medical education systems.

Finally, in the face of the globalization of medical education, we must not unreflectively assume that educational practices in the West are the best. While maintaining awareness of best practices globally, we also have to develop a curriculum that respects local cultural values. For instance, from a Confucian perspective, the self is inseparable from one's social role, and such a stance is very unlike those of Western cultures that often separate the personal and professional life (Ho et al. 2011). Thus, there is greater pressure on physicians in East

Asian contexts to conduct themselves well in both their personal and their professional lives. Another Confucian influence to be aware of is family involvement in a patient's medical care, so that we do not teach patient autonomy in classrooms while practicing the opposite at the bedside.

Appendix A

Appendix 4.A. Medical Universities and Colleges in Taiwan.

Year opened	Name	Public/Private
1897	National Taiwan University College of Medicine	Public
1901 (Moved to Taiwan in 1949)	National Defense Medical Center	Public
1954	Kaohsiung Medical University School of Medicine	Private
1958	China Medical University School of Medicine	Private
1960	Chung Shan Medical University School of Medicine	Private
1960	Taipei Medical University School of Medicine	Private
1975	National Yang Ming University School of Medicine	Public
1984	National Cheng Kung University College of Medicine	Public
1987	Chang Gung University College of Medicine	Private
1990	Fu Jen Catholic University College of Medicine	Private
1994	Tzu Chi University College of Medicine	Private
2009	Mackay Medical College	Private
2013	I-Shou University College of Medicine	Private

Appendix B

Appendix 4.B. Comparative Health System Data.

	Taiwan	China	Hong Kong
Physicians (Total)	40,897	2,466,094	13,006
Physicians per 10,000 Population	17.5	18.2	18.1
Doctors of Chinese Medicine (Total)	5,729	293,465	9,372
Doctors of Chinese Medicine per 10,000 Population	2.5	2.2	12.9
Dentists (Total)	12,391	110,974	2.258

(continued)

Appendix 4.B. Comparative Health System Data. *(continued)*

	Taiwan	China	Hong Kong
Dentists per 10,000 Population	5.3	0.8	3.1
Pharmacists (Total)	15,594	363,993	2,127
Pharmacists per 10,000 Population	6.7	2.7	3
Nurses (Total)	117,804	2,244,020	43,698
Nurses per 10,000 Population	50.5	16.6	61
National Health Expenditure as % of GDP	6.62%	5.15%	5.2%
Per Capita National Health Expenditure (PPP Int.$)	2,546	432.3	12,724 (HK$)
Number of Medical Care Facilities (Total)	21,437	954,389	
Number of Beds (Total)	160,900	5,159,889	35,500
Number of Beds per 10,000 Population	69	38	49.6
Number of Registered Medical Personnel in Hospitals and Clinics (Total)	217,781	6,202,858	
Number of Registered Medical Personnel in Hospitals and Clinics per 10,000 Population	93.4	45.8	

Source: Data from Ministry of Health and Welfare 2013.

References

Accreditation Council for Graduate Medical Education. Last accessed June 25, 2016. http://www.acgme.org.

Centers for Disease Control, Republic of China (Taiwan). 2013. SARS 10年—生聚與教訓 [*SARS Shi Nian—Shengju Yu Jiaoxun*] [*A Decade After SARS: Lessons Learned and Preparedness*]. Taipei: Taiwan Centers for Disease Control.

Chan, L. K., Mary S. M. Ip, N. G. Patil, and M. Prosser. 2011. "Learning Needs in a Medical Curriculum in Hong Kong." *Hong Kong Medical Journal* 17 (3): 202–07.

Chan, Wing P., Ting-Yu Wu, Ming-Shium Hsieh, Ting-Ywan Chou, Chih-Shung Wong, Ji-Tseng Fang, Nen-Chung Chang, Chuang-Ye Hong, and Chii-Ruey Tzeng. 2012. "Students' View Upon Graduation: A Survey of Medical Education in Taiwan." *BMC Medical Education* 12: 127.

———. 2013. "Medical Education Reform in Taiwan: Problems and Solutions." *Medical Education* 17 (2): 50–54.

Chang, Deh-Ming [張德明]. 2012. "由四tt的崩解與整建 [You Si Da Jie Kong Tan Yiliao Zhidude Bengjie Yu Zhengjian] [From The Elements are All Vanity: Discussing the Medical System's Disintegration and Renovation]." 健康世界 [*Jiankang Shijie*] [*Health World*] 320: 23–24.

Chao, Li-Yun [趙麗雲]. 2012. "我國護理人力資源管理問題淺析[Wo Guo Huli Renli Ziyuan Guanli Wenti Qianxi] [An Analysis of Our Country's Nursing Human Resources Management]." National Policy Fundation Research Report. Last accessed August 6, 2016. http://www.exam.gov.tw/lp.asp?CtNode=1192&CtUnit=416&BaseDSD=7&mp=3&nowpage =5&pagesize=20.

Chao Yu, Yu-Mei, Yu-Tzu Dai, and Mei-Chang Yeh (余玉眉, 戴玉慈, 張媚). 2010. "我國護理教育、考試制度與專業核心能力—從國際接軌角度探討 [Wo Guo Huli Jiaoyu, Kaoshi Zhidu Yu Zhuanye Hexin Nengli—Cong Guoji Jiegui Jiaodu Tantao] [Perspectives on Nursing Education, Licensing Examinations and Professional Core Competence in Taiwan in the Context of Globalization]." *The Journal of Nursing* 57 (5): 5–11.

Chen, Shun-Sheng [陳順勝]. 2002. "日據前的西方醫療及其對台灣醫學之影響 [Riju Qiande Xifang Yiliao Ji Qi Dui Taiwan Yixue Zhi Yingxiang] [Western Medical History in Taiwan Before Japanese Control Period]." 科技博物 [Keji Bowu] [*Technology Museum Review*] 6 (4): 59–86.

Chen, Wei J., and Tung-Liang Chiang [陳為堅, 江東亮]. 2010. 公共衛生教育與人力現況與展望 [*Gonggong Weisheng Jiaoyu Yu Renli Xiankuang Yu Zhanwang*] [*Public Health Education and Workforce: Current Status and Perspectives*]. Miaoli, Taiwan: National Health Research Institutes.

Chen, Yen-Yuan, Chau-Chung Wu, Hui-Chi Hsu, Tien-Shang Huang, Ming-Ju Wu, Yen-Hsuan Ni, Chia-Der Lin, Hung-Shiee Lai, Kwo-Chang Ueng, Shan-Chwen Chang, Jer-Chia Tsai, Tzong-Shinn Chu, and Pan-Chyr Yang. 2013. "The Postgraduate General Medical Training in Taiwan: Past, Present and Future." *Journal of Medical Education* 17 (2): 80–91.

Chen, Young-Shing [陳永興]. 1997. 臺灣醫療發展史 [*Taiwan Yiliao Fazhan Shi*] [*History of Medical Development in Taiwan*]. Taipei: 月旦 [Yue Dan].

Cheng, Shou-Hsia. 2013. "從內外婦兒「四大皆空」問題談健保與醫療改革 [Cong Neiwai Fu Er 'Si Da Jie Kong' Wenti Tan Jianbao Yu Yiliao Gaige] [From Inside and Out Women and Children, 'The Four Elements are All Vanity,' Problems Discussing Health Insurance and Medical Reforms]." *NTU Alumni Bimonthly* 86: 21–23.

Chiang, Han-Sun [江漢聲]. 2007a. "從現代醫學的播種談臺灣醫學的萌芽[Cong Xiandai Yixuede Bozhong Tan Taiwan Yixuede Mengya] [From the Current Sowing of Seeds in Medical Education, Discussing the Sprouts of Taiwan's Medical Education]." 歷史月刊 [*Lishi Yuekan*] [*History Monthly*] 238: 33–39.

———. 2007b. "無心插柳—近代日本醫學對臺灣醫學的影響 [Wuxin Cha Liu—Jindai Riben Yixue Dui Taiwan Yixuede Yingxiang] [Unintentionally Entering the Willows: The Influnece of Modern Day Japan's Medical Education on Taiwan's Medical Education]." 歷史月刊 [*Lishi Yuekan*] [*History Monthly*] 239: 38–45.

Chiang, Tung-liang (江東亮). 1995. "臺灣地區的醫師人力政策: 1945–1994 [*Taiwan Diqu De Yishi Renli Zhengce: 1945–1994*] [Physician Manpower Policy in Taiwan, 1945–1994]." *Journal of National Public Health Association Republic of China* 14 (5): 383–91.

———. 2003. 醫療保健政策: 臺灣經驗 [*Yiliao Baojian Zhengce: Taiwan Jingyan*] [*Medical Insurance Policies: The Experience in Taiwan*]. 2nd ed. Taipei: 巨流 [Ju Liu].

Chiu, Chiuang-Husan, Linda Gail Arrigo, and Duu-Jian Tsai. 2009. "Historical Context for the Growth of Medical Professionalism and Curriculum Reform in Taiwan." *Kaohsiung Journal of Medical Sciences* 25 (9): 510–14.

Chiu, Jhih-Ling. 2015. "The Influence of Medical Cost Controls Implemented by Taiwan's National Health Insurance Program on Doctor-Patient Relationships." *The International Journal of Health Planning and Management* 30 (1): E31–E41.

Chou, Jen-Yu, Chiung-Hsuan Chiu, Enoch Lai, Duu-Jian Tsai, and Chii-Ruey Tzeng. 2012. "Medical Education in Taiwan." *Medical Teacher* 34: 187–91.

Chu, Tzong-Shinn, Harrison G. Weed, and Pan-Chyr Yang. 2009. "Recommendations for Medical Education in Taiwan." *Journal of the Formosan Medical Association* 108 (11): 830–33.

Dong, Bao-cheng [董保城]. 2013. "國家考試創新猷—臨床技能測驗(OSCE)納入醫師考試 [Guojia Kaoshi Chuangxin You - Linchuang Jineng Ceyan (OSCE) Naru Yishi Kaoshi] [National Exam Innovation Plan—Clinical Skill Exam Integration into the Medical Exam]." *National Examination Forum* 3 (4): 3–15.

Editorial Board of *Medicine Today*. 1987. "杏林論壇：對長庚醫學院的期望[Xinglin Luntan: Dui Zhanggeng Yixueyuande Qiwang] [A Forest of Apricot Trees Forum: Hopes for Chang Gung University Medical School]." 當代醫學[*Dangdai Yixue*] [*Medicine Today*] 168: 764.

Fan, Angela Pei-Chen, Russell O. Kosikb, Thomas Chen-Chia Tsai, Qiaoling Cai, Guo-Tong Xu, Li Guo, Tung-Ping Su, Shuu-Jiun Wang, Allen Wen-Hsiang Chiu, and Qi Chen. 2014. "A Snapshot of the Status of Problem-Based Learning (PBL) in Chinese Medical Schools." *Medical Teacher* 36 (7): 615–20.

Fan, Yen-chiou [范燕秋]. 1999. "臺灣的美援醫療、防癩政策變動與患者人權問題，1945至1960年代 [Taiwan De Meiyuan Yiliao, Fanglai Zhengce Biandong Yu Huanzhe Renquan Wenti, 1945 Zhi 1960 Niandai] [US Aid Medicine, Hansen's Disease Control Policy, and Patients' Rights in Taiwan (1945–1960s)]." *Taiwan Historical Research* 16 (4): 115–60.

———. 2005. 疾病、醫學與殖民現代性：日治台灣醫學史 [*Jibing、Yixue Yu Zhimin Xiandaixing: Rizhi Taiwan Yixue Shi*] [*Disease, Medicine, and Colonial Modernity: Japan-Occupied Era Taiwan Medical History*]. Taipei: 稻鄉 [Dao Xiang].

Fu Jen Catholic University College of Medicine. Last accessed August 7, 2016. http://www.mc.fju.edu.tw/en/html/aboutUs1.html.

Higher Education Evaluation and Accreditation Council of Taiwan. 2013. *HEEACT 2012 Annual Report*. Taipei: HEEACT.

Ho, Ming-Jung, Kun-Hsing Yu, David Hirsh, Tien-Shang Huang, and Pan-Chyr Yang. 2011. "Does One Size Fit All? Building a Framework for Medical Professionalism." *Academic Medicine* 85: 1407–14.

Ho, Ming-Jung, Kevin Shaw, Tzu-Hung Liu, Jessie Norris, and Yu-Ting Chiu. 2015. "Equal, Global, Local: Discourses in Taiwan's International Medical Graduate Debate." *Medical Education* 49 (1): 48–59.

Hodges, Brian David, Jerry M. Maniate, Maria Athina Martimianakis, Mohammad Alsuwaidan, and Christopher Segouin. 2009. "Cracks and Crevices: Globalization Discourse and Medical Education." *Medical Teacher* 31 (10): 910–17. doi: 10.3109/01421590802534932.

Hsieh, Bor-Shen [謝博生]. 2003. 一般醫學教育：後SARS時代的醫師培育 [*Yiban Yixue Jiaoyu: Hou SARS Shidaide Yishi Peiyu*] [*General Medical Education: The Post-SARS Era Doctor Training*]. Taipei: 國立臺灣大學醫學院出版 [Guoli Taiwan Daxue Yixueyuan Chuban] [National Taiwan University College of Medicine].

———. 2004. 現代醫學在臺灣：臺灣醫學會百年見證 [*Xiandai Yixue Zai Taiwan: Taiwan Yixuehui Bainian Jianzheng*] [*Modern Medicine in Taiwan: Taiwan Medical Conference Centennial Testimonial*]. 2nd ed. Taipei: 國立臺灣大學醫學院出版[Guoli Taiwan Daxue Yixueyuan Chuban] [National Taiwan University College of Medicine].

Hu, Linying, Xiuyun Yin, Xiaolei Bao, and Jin-Bao Nie. 2014. "Chinese Physicians' Attitudes Toward an Understanding of Medical Professionalism: Results of a National Survey." *The Journal of Clinical Ethics* 25 (2): 135–47.

Huang, Chung-I, Cathy Wung, and Che-Ming Yang. 2009. "Developing 21st Century Accreditation Standards for Teaching Hospitals: The Taiwan Experience." *BMC Health Services Research* 9: 232.

Humphreys, George H. II. 2008. "An Early Contact Between the Columbia University College of Physicians and Surgeons and National Taiwan University: Two Accounts." In *Health Care and National Development in Taiwan 1950–2000*, edited by J. R. Watt 62–73. New York: ABMAC Foundation.

I-Shou University College of Medicine. 義守大學獲教部核准102學年設立醫學院 [yi shou da xue huo jiao bu he zhun 102xue nian she li yi xue yuan] [I-Shou University was granted permission to establish medical school in 2013]. Last accessed August 7, 2016. http://www.sec.isu.edu.tw/isu_news/Show.asp?SN=2753.

Juang, Young-Ming [莊永明]. 1998. 臺灣醫療史: 以臺大醫院為主軸 [*Taiwan Yiliao Shi: Yi Taida Yiyuan Wei Zhuzhou*] [*Taiwan Medical History: National Taiwan University Hospital as the Principle Axis*]. Taipei: Yuan-Liou 遠流.

Lai, Chi-Wan. 2009. "Experiences of Accreditation of Medical Education in Taiwan." *Journal of Educational Evaluation for Health Professions* 6: 2.

Lee, Fa-Yauh, Ying-Ying Yang, Hui-Chi Hsu, Chiao-Lin Chuang, Wei-Shin Lee, Ching-Chih Chang, Chia-Chang Huang, Jaw-Wen Chen, Hao-Min Cheng, and Tjin-Shing Jap. 2011. "Clinical Instructors' Perception of a Faculty Development Programme Promoting Postgraduate Year-1 (PGY1) Residents' ACGME Six Core Competencies: A 2-Year Study." *BMJ Open* 1: e000200.

Lee, Robert M. K. W., and Chiu-Yin Kwan. 1997. "The Use of Problem-Based Learning in Medical Education." *Journal of Medical Education* 1 (2): 149–57.

Lin, Chi-Wei, Tsuen-Chiuan Tsai, Cheuk-Kwan Sun, Der-Fang Chen, and Keh-Min Liu. 2013. "Power of the Policy: How the Announcement of High-Stakes Clinical Examination Altered OSCE Implementation at Institutional Level." *BMC Medical Education* 13: 8.

Lin, Pen-Hsuan [林本炫]. 2006. "我國私立大學的設立、經營和合併問題 [*Woguo Sili Daxuede Sheli, Jingying He Hebing Wenti*] [The Foundation, Operation, and Mergence of Private Universities in Taiwan]." *Formosan Education and Society* 10: 65–92.

Lin, Yu-Chih, Yu-Sheng Huang, Chung-Sheng Lai, Jeng-Hsien Yen, and Wen-Chan Tsai. 2009. "Problem-Based Learning Curriculum in Medical Education at Kaohsiung Medical University." *The Kaohsiung Journal of Medical Sciences* 25 (5): 264–70.

Liu, Ching-Kuan. 2013. "Progress of Medical Education in Kauhsiung Medical University." Paper presented at Medical Education in Taiwan: Past and Future, Taipei, Taiwan, April 13.

Liu, Hsin-Chen. 2011. "The Rise of Private Higher Education in Taiwan." Presented at the International Conference on "Innovation in Teaching, Research and Higher Education," Ho Chi Minh City, Vietnam, July 14–15.

Liu, Michael Shi-yung [劉士永]. 1997. "一九三O年代以前臺灣醫學的特質 [*Yijiusanling Niandai Yiqian Taiwan Yixuede Tezhi*] [Characteristics of Taiwanese Medicine Under Japanese Rule Before the 1930s]." 中央研究院臺灣史研究所[*Zhongyang Yanjiuyuan Taiwan Shi Yanjiusuo*] [*Taiwan Historical Research*] 4 (1): 97–148.

———. 2004. "醫療、疾病與台灣社會的近代醫療性格 [*Yi liao、Jibing Yu Taiwan Shehuide Jindai Yiliao Xingge*] [Medical Treatment, Diseases, and Taiwanese Society's Contemporary Medical Character]." 歷史月刊 [*Lishi Yuekan*] [*History Monthly*] 201: 92–100.

———. 2009. *Prescribing Colonization: The Role of Medical Practices and Policies in Japan-Ruled Taiwan, 1895–1945*. Ann Arbor, MI: The Association for Asian Studies.

Lo, Ming-cheng. 2002. *Doctors Within Borders: Profession, Ethnicity, and Modernity in Colonial Taiwan*. Berkeley: University of California Press.

Lo, Tzu Huan. 2008. "ABMAC and Professional Nursing in Taiwan." In *Health Care and National Development in Taiwan 1950–2000*, edited by John R. Watt, 105–121. New York: ABMAC Foundation.

Ministry of Health and Welfare. 2013. Taiwan Public Health Report 2012. Taipei: Ministry of Health and Welfare.

———. 2014. "教學醫院教學費用補助計畫申請作業要點 [Jiaoxue Yiyuan Jiaoxue Feiyong Buzhu Jihua Shenqing Zuoye Yaodian] [Education in Hospitals and Education Expenditures Subsidy Plan Application Tasks Summary]." Last accessed August 7, 2016. http://www.mohw.gov.tw/cht/DOMA/DM1_P.aspx?f_list_no=608&fod_list_no=983&doc_no=1928.

Stevens, Fred C. J., and Jacqueline D. Simmonds Goulbourne. 2012. "Globalization and the Modernization of Medical Education." *Medical Teacher* 34 (10): e684–e689.

Sun, Lucia, Melody Ho, and Derhan Chen. 2013. "The Performance Evaluation on the Electronic Medical Records Project of the Health-Care Systems: A Case Study from the National Audit Office of the Republic of China, Taiwan." *The Current Global Trends* 2 (1): 15–22.

Sytwu, Huey-Kang. 2013. "National Defense Medical Center: A School of 111 Years History." Paper presented at Medical Education in Taiwan: Past and Future, Taipei, Taiwan, April 13.

Taiwan Sheng Xingzheng Zhangguan Gongshu Tongjishi [臺灣省行政長官公署統計室] [Statistics Office for Taiwan Province Magistrate's Government Office]. 1946. 臺灣省五十一年來統計提要 [*Taiwan Sheng Wushiyi Nian Lai Tongji Tiyao*] [*Taiwan Province Year 51 Statistics Summary*]. Taipei: 臺灣省行政長官公署統計室 [Taiwan Sheng Xingzheng Zhangguan Gongshu Tongjishi] [Statistics Office for Taiwan Province Magistrate's Government Office].

Tang, G. 2001. "Quality Assurance of Problem-Based Learning (PBL): The Hong Kong Experience." *Annals, Academy of Medicine, Singapore* 30 (4): 363–65.

Tsai, Duu-Jian. 2008. "Community-Oriented Curriculum Design for Medical Humanities." *Kaohsiung Journal of Medical Sciences* 24 (7): 373–79.

———, ed. 2009. 一個醫師的時代見證：施純仁回憶錄 [*Yige Yishide Shidai Jianzheng: Shi Chun Ren Huiyilu*] [*A Testimontial of One Doctor's Era: A Memoir Bestowing Pure Humaneness*]. Taipei: 記憶工程 [Jiyi Gongcheng].

Tsai, Shih-Li, Ming-Jung Ho, David Hirsh, and David E. Kern. 2012. "Defiance, Compliance, or Alliance? How We Developed a Medical Professionalism Curriculum That Deliberately Connects to Cultural Context." *Medical Teacher* 34 (8): 614–17.

Tsou, Kuo-Inn, Shu-Ling Cho, Chaou-Shune Lin, Leticia B. Sy, Li-King Yang, Ting-Ywan Choua, and Han-Sun Chiang. 2009. "Short-Term Outcomes of a Near-Full PBL Curriculum in a New Taiwan Medical School." *The Kaohsiung Journal of Medical Sciences* 25 (5): 282–93.

Tzu Chi University College of Medicine. "Our Philosophy." Last accessed August 7, 2016. http://eng.tcu.edu.tw/academics/college-of-medicine/#tab-id-1.

Wang, Li-yun. 1996. "Higher Educational Expansion in Taiwan from 1950 to 1994: Patterns and Explanations." Paper presented at the Annual Meeting of the Association for the Study of Higher Education, Memphis, TN, October 31–November 3.

Watt, John R., ed. 2008. *Health Care and National Development in Taiwan 1950–2000*. New York: The ABMAC Foundation.

Xiong, Bing-Zhen, Tung-Liang Chiang, and Li-Jung Cheng. 1990. *The Reminiscenes of Dr. Huo-Yao Wei*. Taipei: Academia Sinica.

Yang, Chao-hsiang. 2007. "中華民國私校教育現況與發展趨勢 [Zhonghua Minguo Sixiao Jiaoyu Xiankuang Yu Fazhan Qushi] [Republic of China Private School Education Current Circumstances and Development Trends]." National Policy Fundation Research Report. Last accessed June 25, 2016. http://www.npf.org.tw/2/3678.

Yang, Tsui-Hua (楊翠華). 2008. "美援對台灣的衛生計畫與醫療體制之形塑 [Meiyuan Dui Taiwande Weishengjihua Yu Yiliao Tizhi Zhi Xingsu] [US Aid in the Formation of Health Planning and Medical System in Taiwan]." *Bulletin of the Institute of Modern History Academia Sinica* 62: 91–139.

Yao, Jen-to. 2003. "Making the Healthy Colonised: Colonial Bodies, Colonial Medicine and Colonial Doctors." Paper presented at 殖民現代性與身體建構小型討論會[Zhimin Xiandaixing Yu Shenti Jiangou Xiaoxing Taolunhui] [Colonial Modernity and Construction of Bodies Small Scale Discussion Forum], Taichung, Tunghai University Department of Sociology, March 22.

Yeh, Yun-Wen (葉永文). 2003. "日據時期台灣的醫政關係 [Rijushiqi Taiwande Yizheng Guanxi] [Medical and Politics of Taiwan During Japanese Occupation]." *Formosan Journal of Medical Humanities* 4 (1–2): 48–68.

———. 2004. "戰後台灣的醫政關係(1945–1975): 弱勢統治與強勢統治的分析 [Zhanhou Taiwande Yizheng Guanxi (1945–1975): Ruoshi Tongzhi Yu Qiangshi Tongzhide Fenxi] [The Relationship Between Medicine and Politics in Postwar Taiwan (1945–1975): An Analysis of Weak Government and Strong Government]." *Social Policy & Social Work* 8 (2): 1–38.

5 A Brief History of Medical Education in Hong Kong

Gabriel M. Leung and N. G. (Niv) Patil

THE DEVELOPMENT OF medical education, and more generally Western medicine, in what has now come to be known as the Greater China region is an instructive story intertwined with colonialism, civil strife, revolutions, and more recently, macroeconomic development and accompanying social change. As Rudolf Virchow put it, "politics is nothing else but medicine on a large scale" (Friedlander 2005). Of course, the converse is even truer, as this chapter illustrates. As such, the historically distinct, parallel evolution of medical education in mainland China, Taiwan, and Hong Kong, which share a common heritage but have traveled down rather different paths in the modern development of health care or medical education, provides useful lessons for anticipating possible consequences of policy and politics.

In this chapter, we will describe how geopolitical events have shaped the very different developmental pathways of Western allopathic medical education in the three main political entities in the region. We focus on the case of Hong Kong, a former British colony that has become a Special Administrative Region of mainland China. As it turned out, Hong Kong's history was equivalent to that of a single institution, the Li Ka Shing Faculty of Medicine of the University of Hong Kong (founded as the Hong Kong College of Medicine for Chinese), until the mid-1970s when a second medical school was commissioned at the Chinese University of Hong Kong. Mainland China and Taiwan are considered in depth in chapters 3 and 4 of the present volume, respectively.

The Arrival of Western Medicine

Divergent Foreign Influences in Greater China

Whereas mainland China has practiced traditional medicine for millenniums, modern methods from the West were introduced to the country along trade and missionary routes only since the nineteenth century in the major coastal cities. Protestant medical missionaries, heralded by the earlier arrival of Robert Morrison of the London Missionary Society in Canton (Guangzhou) in 1807, started to work in the country from the 1830s onward. These were mostly men from Britain and America, such as Peter Parker, Benjamin Hobson, and William Lockhart. The London Missionary Society's hospital in Peking, among dozens of hospitals all over the country, was founded by Lockhart in 1861 and became the basis on which Peking Union Medical College (PUMC) was built (Paterson 1987). PUMC in the capital was the defining landmark established in 1917 by the Rockefeller Foundation and nurtured by its spinoff, the China Medical Board, not long after the modern republic was founded. With the later birth of the People's Republic in 1949, the development of medical education naturally fell under the influence of the prevailing Soviet model until the "reform and opening up" movement launched by Deng Xiaoping in 1979, when Anglo-American influences began to return (see chapter 3 of the present volume).

On the other side of the Taiwan Strait off the mainland, successive European colonial powers had been bringing their respective home influences with them since the seventeenth century, although the German-Japanese model came to predominate during the first half of the twentieth century when the island was a Japanese colony and the American system became the primary template after 1949 (see chapter 4 of the present volume).

Hong Kong, by far the smallest of the Greater China trio, took yet a different road. The modern story of Hong Kong began as a product of the Treaty of Nanjing, following the outbreak of the First Opium War. In 1841, it became a British colony (Tsang 2004). With this, the foundation for a thoroughly British influence on the development of health care and associated professional training was firmly laid, and it persists to the present, as it has been only twenty years since the Special Administrative Region's repatriation in 1997. For this reason, the Hong Kong system, unlike those in mainland China and Taiwan, has been modeled exclusively on the British system, and its development closely mirrors the evolution of health care changes in Britain.

Western Medical Beginnings

Having moved to the newly established British colony from the Portuguese colony of Macau, Hobson opened the Medical Missionary Hospital of Hong Kong, the territory's first such facility, in 1843. The hospital operated for exactly a decade, when the second medical superintendent after Hobson packed up for his next assignment in Amoy (Xiamen). For the next twenty years, Hong Kong did not have a Western medical facility that treated the Chinese masses. The Government Civil Hospital mostly cared for the expatriate community and Chinese government servants. Then, in 1872, Tung Wah Hospital opened its doors, although it offered only traditional Chinese medicine (TCM) at the outset due to the overwhelming preference of the local population at the time.

This hospital was founded by a group of local Chinese elites, and to this day, it remains the leading charity focused on health care, education, and elderly services.

It would be another fifteen years before the Alice Memorial Hospital was commissioned. There were various dispensaries and clinics along the way, but none lasted. After a six-year gestation period, the project received its final push from Ho Kai, son of a Chinese pastor, an Aberdonian medical graduate, and a barrister of Lincoln's Inn who recently returned from his studies. The original quartet of clinical staff comprised Patrick Manson, William Hartigan, William Young, and Gregory Jordan, as well as James Cantlie and John Bell, both of whom were recruited later, when the hospital started taking in new patients.

Hong Kong College of Medicine: A Medical School for Chinese

Barely six months after the Alice Memorial Hospital opened, Manson and the other medical men (including Ho Kai, but not William Young), in conjunction with John Chalmers of the London Missionary Society and Frederick Stewart, a school master turned senior civil servant, proceeded to realize the next step of their dream—the establishment of a medical school. The idea of having a local school producing doctors, however, did not arise impulsively. The idea had, in fact, developed in parallel to the planning of the Alice Memorial Hospital. In his 1887 inaugural speech as founding Dean of the Hong Kong College of Medicine for Chinese, Manson emphatically stated that it was to be a school for the whole of China:

> I can conceive no grander position or opportunity for any man to have than that we offer to each of our students. At his back the whole of European science, before him 300,000,000 to whom to give it. Such a position must fire the ambition of some of them. It is most strange that no great man, or great men, have arisen for this work. He, and they, will come. The old Greek cities used to boast of their great men and claim them with jealous care. Let us hope that in the new and greater China of the future, when the learned dispute of their great men, not a few may be claimed for Hongkong and for the School to-day inaugurated.
>
> And when these reforms are effected and changes made, what to us Europeans will be the consequences? Politically over three hundred million of the most industrious, thrifty, persevering, homogeneous, physically adaptable, clever people, at present hardly a cipher in political calculations, will be no insignificant factor in the combinations of the future. Their numbers, no longer kept under by preventable disease, civil wars, infanticide, or polygamy, will rapidly increase and they will expand in all directions. Perhaps the deadly upas tree of opium will by that time have been uprooted. Minor peoples, Annamites, Siamese, Malays, will go down before them or be absorbed by them. A great homogeneous Chinese-speaking nation will spread from

Siberia to Australia. It requires little of the prophetic to foresee this. The process has already commenced. In those days wise men will again come from the East. The people who gave us the invention of printing will give yet other peaceful and useful arts; the first to use gunpowder will not be backward in the art of war; the discoverers of inoculation will add again to the prevention and cure of disease. Those hundreds of millions will double the recruiting ground of science and may yet give back to Europe more than they got. It seems to me sometimes that we are teaching the Chinese to beat ourselves (Manson 1888, 68–72).

While the founding of the college, and later of the University of Hong Kong, undoubtedly had a strong imperial undertone, it is noteworthy that, in this speech, Manson already envisioned the asymmetry of the relationship whereby this venture could "give back to Europe more than they got." This debate about the role, form, and value of imperialism would recur time and again throughout the school's several existential crises of periodic budgetary shortfalls and even discussions of whether the school should close its doors until the end of the Second World War.

It is generally acknowledged that Boji Medical School, the forerunner of present-day Sun Yat-Sen University Zhongshan School of Medicine, which was founded in 1866, was the first school of Western medicine in China. The now defunct Peiyang (or Bei Yang) Medical College based in Tianjin, which was first inaugurated as the Viceroy's Hospital Medical School in 1881 by the late Qing high official Li Hung-Chang to train military surgeons, was the second institution of Western medical learning in the country (Wu 1995). The Hong Kong College of Medicine for Chinese (omitting "for Chinese" in its name from 1907 onward) was thus actually the third such establishment chronologically. Nonetheless, Manson's inaugural speech contains a strong sense of the importance of history and the vision that the college was to become a model for the rest of the country.

The first two graduates from the Hong Kong Medical College were Sun Yat-Sen, revolutionary hero and acknowledged founding father of modern China, and Kong Ying-Wa in 1892. The editors of *The Lancet* declared "sincere satisfaction" with this first success of the medical education experiment in Hong Kong and praised the college's role as an instrument through which "science enters [China] like a beam of pure sunlight, and with it truth" (*The Lancet* Editors 1892, 621). It is worth noting the imperial imagery of the college as a beacon of light in Asia, which in fact coincided with Governor Frederick Lugard's ideals that led him to establish the University of Hong Kong two decades later. Cecil Clementi, who later also became governor, summed it up best in the final stanza of the university's anthem, which he penned to be sung at the opening ceremony:

Dei
Semper auxilio novum
Splendeat sapientia
Lumen ex Oriente!
[By God's grace,
May the new light of wisdom
Ever shine out
From the East!] (Clementi 1892)

The Transition to the Faculty of Medicine, University of Hong Kong (1887–1911)

The Hong Kong College of Medicine operated on a threadbare model throughout its independent existence (Cunich and Cowell 2012). It did not possess its own premises, although not for lack of trying and a number of near misses. Clinical instruction took place mostly in the Alice Memorial Hospital and later the Nethersole and Tung Wah Hospitals. It relied almost exclusively on what we would today call "honorary teachers," practitioners who took time out from their private practice to give lessons out of a sense of civic duty. This approach was quintessentially British in origin in that it was an apprenticeship model in which practitioners in an existing hospital formed the core of the teaching organization (Evans 1987). In fact, an important proportion of clinical teaching continues today to be delivered by honorary staff outside of the employ of the medical school.

Unlike the better British institutions of the time, however, the college had had virtually no research to speak of throughout its entire existence or, for that matter, during the early years in the careers of any of its faculty members (Evans 1987, 63). Patrick Manson, who was widely credited with having worked out the vector-borne transmission mode of filariasis and, in so doing, paving the way for Ronald Ross's Nobel Prize on deciphering the malaria cycle years later (Chernin 1983), was a notable exception, although during his two-year affiliation with the college, he did not carry out experiments on site.

The transition from an independent college to the Faculty of Medicine at the University of Hong Kong did not happen as seamlessly as might be imagined. The process was subject to many negotiated compromises and took a long while to complete. In fact, for five or six years the two entities coexisted.

Of particular note, one immediate advantage associated with becoming part of a formal university concerned licensure, as graduates could now acquire professional certification that was recognized by both the Medical Council of Hong Kong and the UK General Medical Council, and which had been previously unattainable for almost a quarter of a century (Evans 1987, 60).

Stuttering Growth for the Faculty of Medicine (1911–1940)

"Failure to thrive," which is a medical term to describe a struggling child starved of nutrition, can aptly summarize the Faculty of Medicine's first decade and a half. It needed to transition from a virtual establishment of part-time teachers to a permanent staff whose primary duty was to fashion and maintain a degree program. Given the newfound accreditation by the UK General Medical Council, this obligation was all the more pressing in the face of the rapidly changing landscape of medical education back in Britain (as indeed in the newly formed republic on the Chinese mainland), specifically the 1913 Royal Commission on University Education, which recommended wholesale, resource-intensive infrastructural improvements to the undergraduate learning experience. The ripples of the 1910 Flexner Report in the United States were very much felt and were in many ways reflected in the Royal Commission's work.

Unfortunately, the university's finances came perilously close to a precipice just as the need for institutional funds was at its most acute. Due to a lack of proper financial planning, lax oversight, and serious mismanagement, the University Court had to reject the 1919–1920 accounts, leading to a government enquiry and subsequent bailout.

At the eleventh hour, the New York-based Rockefeller Foundation came to the rescue, offering a substantial endowment for three key professorships in medicine, surgery, and obstetrics. This source of funding became the only fiscal lifeline, as the colonial government refused to supply additional resources. The Rockefeller Foundation had been exceptionally generous, especially when it wisely decided to release the university from the original conditions attached to the grant that the government refused to consider. These conditions concerned designating the Government Civil Hospital for university purposes, the building of a medical student residence, and guaranteed subvention amounts.

Interestingly, although the first condition initially specified by Richard Pearce, Rockefeller's director of medical education, was never fulfilled, within fifteen years of the formal acceptance of the endowment in 1922, a new hospital replacing the functions of the Government Civil Hospital (Queen Mary Hospital) became the de facto main teaching hospital affiliated with the Faculty of Medicine, and it has remained so through the present day.

During this period, the Faculty of Medicine continued to produce a steady stream of fewer than twenty graduates annually, although even at this level, there were worries about "supersaturating the local market" (Evans 1987, 73) and bringing about medical unemployment, or at least underemployment. This was compounded by the fact that more than a few of the students came from different parts of the mainland and from Southeast Asia. The atmosphere in government circles became so toxic that some began to question whether the university operated *for* Hong Kong or merely *in* Hong Kong. If the latter was the case, then perhaps the home government in London should have been footing the bill. On the other hand, the percentage of Colonial Office government officials who still believed that the university was "probably our best form of propaganda in China" continued to dwindle through the 1920s and 1930s (ibid., 243). All this culminated in the commissioning of the so-called "1937 Committee," whose unfriendly conclusions questioned the purpose of the university and criticized its listless drift.

In response, then Vice Chancellor and Professor of Physiology Lindsay Ride recommended to the 1937 Committee to reconstitute the College of Medicine as an independent entity that would be affiliated with the university, just as the London hospital-based medical schools were separate organizations that had retained ties with the University of London. This never came to be. Instead, incoming Vice Chancellor Duncan Sloss set up a development committee at the university to deal with the fallout arising from the work of the government-appointed 1937 Committee. A "1939 Report" with much more constructive (albeit similar) viewpoints was eventually produced that proved instrumental in cushioning the negative impact of the earlier document. However, none of this quite compared with the devastating impact of the looming Second World War.

War in the Pacific Theater and its Aftermath (1941–1949)

Christmas Day of 1941 brought three years and eight months of occupation by the Japanese, and with it, all operations of the University came to a full stop. Brave faculty members and university supporters, however, expended heroic efforts while interned in Stanley Prison, where several university senate meetings were even held. By the end of 1942, 140 medical students dispersed to six schools in the southwestern provinces of "Free China" to continue their studies, just as the Faculty of Medicine hosted Lingnan medical students when their school had to close earlier during the war. Gordon King, Dean and Professor of Obstetrics, wrote to the General Medical Council from Chongqing while in exile, successfully petitioning the granting of professional recognition to these wartime studies (Matthews and Cheung 1998).

On the institutional front, with the war over, Christopher Cox was tasked by the Secretary of State for the Colonies, Arthur Creech-Jones, to convene a committee to consider the university's strategic future and finances. Although never published, the Cox Report recommended continuance of the University of Hong Kong to serve Hong Kong's people primarily, which was the first articulation of a reorientation toward local needs and a marked departure from the original Lugardian imperialistic aims. Duncan Sloss, who oversaw the university through the war until 1949, increasingly came to the same view as Manson's inauguration address had foreshadowed at the founding of the college some sixty years prior. Sloss wanted to position the university as a cultural interlocutor between East and West with bilateral flow and exchanges, which also reflected the general shift in thinking as a result of the waning influence of the British Empire and its diminished and revised role in the colonies and the wider world following conclusion of World War II (Matthews and Cheung 1998, 436).

Momentum started to build, and the Faculty of Medicine and the University of Hong Kong slowly began to function again from around 1948 onward, with its financial position much improved.

Progressing to Modernity

The Postwar Decades (1950–1980)

The Cox Report's strategic refocus on local welfare presaged impending massive socio-demographic and economic changes Hong Kong was about to face during the three postwar decades. Much of the present Hong Kong population was formed by migration from the mainland after the People's Republic was founded in 1949. The local population swelled from 600,000 just after the war ended to 2 million by 1950 and to 2.5 million five years after that (Matthews and Cheung 1998, 167). Unlike previous waves of migration, virtually all of these new Hongkongers would stay, given the difficulties of crossing the border through the Korean War embargo and the Cold War, the strife caused by the Great Famine and the Cultural Revolution in mainland China, and the pull of imminent economic takeoff in Hong Kong. As such, along with rapid economic growth, a modern welfare state began. Murray MacLehose's decade of governorship throughout the 1970s was emblematic of a large crescendo in spending, first on housing, education, and social protection, and finally on health care.

In 1950, the Inter-University Council for Higher Education in the Colonies endorsed Cox's recommendations for growth with greater financial commitment during a visit to Hong Kong by representatives Mouat Jones and Walter Adams. Three years later, Governor Alexander Grantham asked Ivor Jennings, the Vice Chancellor of Celyon, and Douglas Logan, the Principal of the University of London, to "examine and make recommendations on the constitution, function and financial requirements of the University in the light of the Cox and Mouat Jones/Adams Reports and any Reports and developments since" (Evans 1987, 88).

Jennings and Logan were unsparing in their criticism of the Faculty of Medicine's laboratories and teaching facilities for being ill-housed and understaffed. Regarding clinical teaching, the report was damning of government in the lack of coordination between the faculty and Queen Mary Hospital. The crux of the matter concerned ownership of and responsibility for beds. At Tsan Yuk Hospital, the Professor of Obstetrics and Gynecology had total control at the maternity facility, as should be preferred, while at Queen Mary Hospital, fewer than half of the beds were managed by the university itself, with the majority of beds being managed by government staff.

This troubled relationship has continued to plague clinical teaching and services to this day. In fact, it has been part of the justification for the Faculty of Medicine's very recent forays into projects at HKU-Shenzhen Hospital and at Gleneagles Hospital.

Of the three postwar reports in quick succession, the Jennings/Logan Report had the most direct and largest impact on the development of the Faculty of Medicine over the next few decades in terms of rapidly scaling up and broadening the scope of coverage to a wider range of specialties. As a result, the modern faculty began to take shape with major infrastructural improvements that laid the groundwork for its sterling reputation today (Evans 1987).

A New Sister School (1974–1981)

The history of medical education in Hong Kong had so far necessarily been equivalent to the development of the one and only medical school at that time. This changed, however, in 1974 when the Legislative Council approved to commission a second medical school at the Chinese University of Hong Kong. The first class was admitted in 1981, almost a century after the Hong Kong College of Medicine for Chinese formally registered its inaugural cohort. The motivation for a new medical school stemmed from MacLehose's rapid expansion of the modern welfare state. Landmark breakthrough social policies—such as nine years of free education, the massive ten-year scaling up of public housing construction, the introduction of a new subsidized home ownership scheme for the sandwich class, and the establishment of the Comprehensive Social Security Assistance program—were launched during his decade in office. On the health care front, there was a concomitant need to produce more doctors to staff the new hospitals being built at the time. The government estimated at the time that one hundred additional doctors would be required every year (Li 1978). By the year the new school took in its first students, the population reached 5.1 million. To encourage competition, it was believed that a second medical school should be preferred over simply allocating the extra student places to the one and only preexisting school, which was already admitting 150 students per year. Moreover, the Chinese University of Hong Kong had a geographical advantage in that it is situated in Shatin, which was to become Hong Kong's first "new town" in the New Territories, which were once exclusively rural. Currently, almost one in ten Hongkongers lives in Shatin. This was, and continues to be, where the demand for new doctors would be most acute, compared to the much less densely populated Hong Kong Island, where the University of Hong Kong is based.

Interestingly, the Vice-chancellor of the Chinese University of Hong Kong, Choh-Ming Li, declared that this new medical program aimed "to produce a new breed of doctors for Hong Kong who are willing to spend their entire career in the service of the [government] Medical and Health Department or the University instead of entering private practice after biding their time in hospital posts for a limited period" (ibid., 16). Perhaps unsurprisingly, such noble aspirations never came to pass. Nevertheless, the Chinese University of Hong Kong has produced many high quality graduates, very much comparable to those of the University of Hong Kong.

A Postgraduate Academy (1979–1993)

So far, we have restricted the discussion to undergraduate medical education. However, the professional requirements of a modern doctor have long evolved into a learning continuum including a structured postgraduate specialty (and possibly subspecialty) training, lifelong continuous professional development, and most recently, even periodic revalidation in some advanced economies.

Prior to the establishment of the Hong Kong Academy of Medicine in 1993, Hong Kong had always relied on English, Scottish, or more recently, Australian royal colleges for external validation and certification of all postgraduate specialty programs. However, it was recognized very early on, during the 1970s in fact, that postgraduate specialty accreditation should be systematized and formally regulated by a local authority. The initial discussions revolved around adding a "specialist register" to be maintained by the Medical Council of Hong Kong. In turn, the council formed the "Working Party on a Specialist Register for Hong Kong" in 1979, which made a report three years later. In response to the report's recommendations, a joint committee of the Hong Kong Medical Association and British Medical Association (Hong Kong Branch) was instituted in 1983. It concluded that a specialist register per se would do little to improve medical care unless supported by a new governing body and more generally improved facilities and provisions for specialist training.

Closely following the joint committee report in 1984, another major motivation for an independent postgraduate training body arose from the signing of the Sino-British Joint Declaration for Hong Kong's repatriation. The firm prospect of Chinese resumption of sovereignty brought home the realization that reliance on foreign accreditation bodies would no longer be tenable after 1997. On the other hand, there was, and still is, no parallel system on the mainland to which the local medical community could consider switching. Therefore, Hong Kong would need to administer its own system, (ideally both externally benchmarked and reciprocally recognized) for specialty training, examination, and accreditation.

Thirdly, there was a severe lack of structured, supervised training programs across most specialties that were available domestically. Those who had wished for better postgraduate opportunities would typically apply overseas for fellowship posts.

Keith Halnan, a British expert in postgraduate medical training from the Hammersmith Hospital in London, was enlisted to submit recommendations by chairing the Working Party on Postgraduate Medical Education and Training in 1988. The report was unanimously supported by all vested parties and the medical community at large. Halnan passed the baton for implementation to David Todd, a local medical doyen and Professor of Medicine at the University of Hong Kong. Todd rallied a roll call of "who's who" of medical men and women, implemented the recommendations of the Halnan report (although not without the usual dose of controversies associated with disrupting the status quo), and led the creation of the Hong Kong Academy of Medicine within four short years. The Academy was inaugurated in 1993 with twelve founding colleges, and it has since added three more colleges that were established subsequently.

Future Possibilities (2015–Present)

As the inaugural Halnan lecturer,[1] David Todd delivered the pensively entitled lecture "Medicine—*quo vadis*?"—in other words, "Where is medicine going?" The final section here reassesses this question for medical education specifically, with the benefit of the hindsight of the history as described above.

Hong Kong started offering institutionalized Western medicine in 1843, led by expatriate missionaries. The British system of medical education, and of healthcare more generally, had left indelible imprints on how local institutions were run. Teachers and especially those in leadership positions had largely been imported from Britain and, to a lesser extent, elsewhere in the Commonwealth. Specialist accreditation was granted by and curriculums were benchmarked against the British and Commonwealth royal colleges. Over time, with socioeconomic development, in situ expertise and capacity grew, thus allowing Hong Kong to pursue localization in all aspects of the medical system. A firm push was given by the Sino-British Joint Declaration of 1984, which laid out the negotiated steps for the return of sovereignty from the former colonial power to the motherland, in that the number of expatriates started to dwindle and the eventuality of integration with the mainland began to be recognized. The localization process of institutions and personnel (although not of ethos or character of systems) was finally complete with the founding of the Hong Kong Academy of Medicine in 1993, exactly 150 years after Benjamin Hobson opened the Medical Missionary Hospital of Hong Kong. This period almost completely overlaps with that of the British colonial administration. For this reason, the template for the various component parts of medical education would be British in origin, or more precisely English (given the recent divergence of the Welsh and Scottish systems since devolution of authority from Westminster).

As soon as localization had been fully achieved and the repatriation to Chinese sovereignty came to pass, the thoroughly British-based system started to turn inward, however. Students who enrolled in previously recognized

Commonwealth medical schools after 1997 could no longer qualify without sitting for the licensing examination of the Medical Council of Hong Kong (Licentiate Committee of the Medical Council of Hong Kong 2014). The pass rate of this three-part examination hovered around 10 percent until a tentative upturn in the past couple of years. This contrasts with progressively more liberal attitudes toward international medical graduates in the United Kingdom (General Medical Council 2014), Australia (Australian Medical Council Limited 2014), and Singapore (Singapore Medical Council 2014), especially those who are already accredited specialists in their countries of origin and would be admitted through credentialing of competencies achieved. On the postgraduate training front, the constituent colleges of the Hong Kong Academy of Medicine differ in the latitude they allow in recognizing foreign medical experience, sometimes even for training offered by the very English or Australian royal colleges with which Hong Kong counterparts still hold joint examinations.

On the other hand, Hong Kong has not opened up to mainland Chinese graduates, which is perhaps more understandable given China's regional disparities in the quality of medical education and its sheer overwhelming size. This leaves the two local medical schools to form a de facto duopoly on the pool of academic medical expertise. Achieving a flow of new ideas in or out of the local system has therefore become harder than it used to be. This situation has never happened before, and whether Hong Kong can continue to excel with its small population of just over seven million has been called into question. Concomitantly, there is a widely acknowledged shortage of medical and, for that matter, nursing personnel, and this situation is predicted to persist for the foreseeable future. There were, as of 2012, 1.82 doctors and 5.46 nurses per 1,000 population, compared to 3.15 and 8.17 for OECD (the Organization for Economic Cooperation and Development) countries (see Table 5.1).

Given Hong Kong's mode of economic development through free trade, which has, in fact, been consistently ranked the world's freest economy by the US-based Heritage Foundation for twenty consecutive years (Heritage Foundation 2014), and given the fact that today's local economy no longer manufactures or trades in goods but relies predominantly on services (92.9 percent as of 2013 [Hong Kong Census and Statistics Department 2015]), the fact that the city's medical economy is relatively closed in terms of healthcare personnel might be surprising (although it is not closed in terms of medical equipment, devices, pharmaceuticals, or goods in general). In comparison to the other professions, medicine is arguably the least welcoming of foreign graduates, many of whom are in fact indigenous Hongkongers who have studied abroad and would like to return home to practice medicine. On the demand side, there is a crescendo of voices arguing against "medical tourists" (mostly from the mainland) taking up scarce healthcare human resources and displacing locals who are less willing or able to pay for private services. This is in stark contrast to the proactive, wholesale

Table 5.1. A Comparison of Human Resources for Health, 2012.

	No. of doctors	No. of nurses	No. of traditional medicine practitioners
	(per 1,000 population)		
OECD average	3.15	8.17	
China	1.49	1.84	0.27
Hong Kong	1.82	6.74	1.30
Japan	2.29	10.54	
Singapore	1.58	6.50	0.52
South Korea	2.08	4.84	
Taiwan	1.76	5.90	0.25
United Kingdom	2.75	8.21	
United States	2.46	11.14	

Sources: For OECD average, Japan, South Korea, and United Kingdom, data from Organisation for Economic Co-Operation and Development 2014. For China, data from National Health and Family Planning Commission of the People's Republic of China 2013. For Hong Kong, data from Hong Kong Census and Statistics Department 2014. For Singapore, data from Singapore Medical Council (2013), Singapore Nursing Board 2013, and Singapore Traditional Chinese Medicine Practitioners Board 2012. For Taiwan, data from Directorate-General of Budget, Accounting and Statistics, Republic of China 2015.

promotion of healthcare services by Singapore and Thailand, who are working to attract foreign patients.

On a more positive note, in addition to its role as the ultimate arbiter of specialist competencies, the Hong Kong Academy of Medicine can serve as a useful intermediary, brokering Western best practices by retaining its connection with the Commonwealth royal colleges and extending its influence into mainland China. Regarding the latter, China has yet to develop a nationwide specialist accreditation system. Currently, such functions are confined within individual institutions and vary between and within provinces. As Hong Kong's business sector has long contributed to the mainland's "reform and opening up" since 1979, brokering financing, legal, and management acumen, its public health care sector too has, in the past decade, served as a useful reference template for the country's ongoing health system reform efforts. Such examples include standardized drug formulary, a centralized regulatory regime for all hospitals modeled on the Hong Kong's Hospital Authority. Similarly, if the Hong Kong Academy of Medicine can realize some of the pilot projects already underway in the last few years by certain specialty colleges nationwide and increase their scale, the potential for the Hong Kong medical community to grow in stature and to influence the course of the medical system for the whole country would be enormous.

At the undergraduate level, local schools of medicine should identify unique niche areas in which they could grow to lead the country and the ASEAN (Association of Southeast Asian Nations) region. Such areas may include, among others, building a contextually relevant collaborative problem-based learning case bank, sharing pedagogical techniques using English as the medium of instruction, defining and following competency-driven instructional approaches, and adapting and brokering innovative curricular solutions with schools in the developing regions of the Western Pacific and Southeast Asia. The East-West Alliance, a network of medical schools[2] that have benefitted from major donations by the Li Ka Shing Foundation, is a potentially powerful example. The China Medical Board is another important philanthropic catalyst that has bound schools and people together and that, throughout its one hundred years of history, has provided critical support to many in the region, including a struggling young University of Hong Kong. Above all, Hong Kong could play a core facilitative role in advancing what Julio Frenk and his collaborators have called "third-generation reforms," which are "systems based to improve the performance of health systems by adapting core professional competencies to specific contexts, while drawing on global knowledge" (Frenk et al. 2010, 6). This makes sense because Hong Kong possesses the necessary competencies, has the understanding of the region as a whole (and of China and Taiwan in particular), and has a long history of deep global engagement, especially with the British Commonwealth.

A case in point concerns the teaching of medical ethics and the humanities. While both local schools have included these subjects in their undergraduate curriculums, further value-added contributions could easily be foreseen. First, the role of the Confucian worldview, vis-à-vis the ethics of a *ren* (仁)-based philosophy (Tao 2006) has so far been less explored in the global literature, let alone applied to any extent anywhere, including in the Greater China region. Second, the disturbing phenomenon of violence against medical workers (「醫患」) on the mainland in recent years screams for an urgent study whose results would be shared with those in training. The anticipated introduction of a master's course in medical ethics and law by the University of Hong Kong's Cambridge-affiliated center and the Chinese University's recent inauguration of its own center could make useful and important contributions toward such a goal. On the other hand, the Medical Council of Hong Kong commended the University of Hong Kong's medical humanities curriculum in particular in its 2014 quinquennial program review. The program is a longitudinal, experiential, and multi-modal curriculum that includes literature, visual arts, and performing and behavioral arts to understand and experience medicine and its meaning to patients, caregivers, and the public.

A potential recent disruptive technological innovation in education is the rise of MOOCs, or massive open online courses. While a sustainable business plan for MOOCs has yet to be fully developed, an added consideration for the Chinese market (and to a lesser extent, other developing Asian markets) concerns penetration and uptake. If the commercial online marketplace bears any indication, providers that may well be household names in the West are often little known or used (and sometimes even blocked) in China. Domestic rivals that show unique local acumen and that have garnered the trust of the authorities prosper over their foreign counterparts. Hong Kong, ever the go-between East and West, can leverage its unique advantages of having an unfettered, highly efficient information technology infrastructure, true bicultural understanding of working in and with the mainland, and world class competencies in medical teaching and learning to deliver added value to this new enterprise.

Developing a new model of truly integrative medicine, that is a mixture of Western methods with traditional Chinese medicine practice, has been an area of intense interest of late. Since 2000, the government has required Chinese medicine practitioners to be registered through a statutory system akin to their allopathic counterparts. The development and marketing of herbal and proprietary Chinese medicinal products similarly need to be vetted and approved. In fact, Hong Kong has long been a stalwart partner of the World Health Organization in pushing the regulatory agenda for traditional medicine of all types at the global level. There are three local Chinese medicine schools, at the University of Hong Kong, the Chinese University of Hong Kong, and Baptist University. There are active plans for a government-supported Chinese medicine hospital to be commissioned during the coming decade. Whereas colonial Hong Kong began with a populace that was deeply mistrustful of Western medicine, present-day Hong Kong is predominantly reliant on Western medicine, although traditional Chinese medicine practitioners have continued to play a complementary role. Rudyard Kipling once wrote, "Oh, East is East and West is West, and never the twain shall meet" (Kipling 1889). Given its unique history, Hong Kong could bring the best of the Western scientific tradition to explore ancient Chinese medical wisdom. Many before have tried, but they have yet to find success. The ultimate prize is still to be claimed.

The list of possibilities is inexhaustible, and crystal ball gazing is a hazardous game. We have merely mentioned a few pertinent examples as a basis for reflection and debate. We have attempted to show the historical nuances of medical education development in the small but pivotal city of Hong Kong compared against the much larger canvases of mainland China and Taiwan. In doing so, we have restricted the discourse to focus on medical education because the development of nursing, public health, and other allied health professional training would require separate treatments to do justice to their equal importance.

Hong Kong has come a long way, from excelling at what Frenk and colleagues call "informative learning" to more recently shaping doctors of the highest moral character through the medical ethics and humanities curriculums and experiential learning outside the classroom. Its next step must be to leap over the chasm of transformative education to produce medical change agents through inculcating system-wide leadership attributes (Frenk et al. 2010, 6, 34). For instance, Hong Kong is uniquely well positioned to become a true pioneer at engineering the birth and development of the new discipline of integrative medicine, bringing out the best of traditional Chinese practice's allopathic methods, given the coexistence of both systems in an advanced society that the world understands and trusts. Similarly, its accreditation system is a good model for the rest of China to emulate and adapt, given the national void at present and the desperate need for the quality assurance demanded by a burgeoning middle class that is the world's largest and most rapidly emerging. Such challenges for transforming systems for health require medical change agents who have distinct leadership qualities and dare to aspire to ambitious goals.

Hong Kong is at a crossroads—it needs to proceed wisely in order to continue leading the region as the circumstances of history have enabled it to do thus far. To succeed, it needs to reinvent systems, innovate at the cutting edge, and integrate further and more deeply with mainland China. It must adhere to its history of open engagement with the world (albeit momentarily interrupted at present) that would allow the rapid spread and adoption of the best ideas from anywhere in real time. Hong Kong should regain its lost confidence that it can lead by welcoming competition and win through expanding and enhancing capacity throughout the entire medical enterprise.

Notes

1. The Halnan Lecture was established, in honor of Professor Sir Keith Halnan, as the Academy's most prestigious named lecture usually delivered at its annual fellowship conferment ceremony.
2. In alphabetic order, as at March 2014, the list includes Alberta, Cambridge, Chinese University of Hong Kong, Hong Kong University, Manitoba, Oxford, Shantou, Stanford, Toronto, UC Berkeley, UCSF, and UMCG.

References

Australian Medical Council Limited. 2014. "Assessment Pathways to Registration for International Medical Graduates." Last accessed June 26, 2016. http://www.amc.org.au/index.php/ass/apo.

Chernin, Eli. 1983. "Sir Patrick Manson's Studies on the Transmission and Biology of Filariasis." *Reviews of Infectious Diseases* 5 (1): 148–66.

Clementi, Cecil. 1892. "University Anthem." Last accessed August 8, 2016. http://100.hku.hk/doc/anthem.pdf.

Cunich, Peter and Christopher Cowell. 2012. *A History of the University of Hong Kong.* Hong Kong: Hong Kong University Press.

Directorate-General of Budget, Accounting and Statistics, Republic of China. 2015. "Taiwan Monthly Bulletin of Statistics (January 2015)." Last accessed November 11, 2015. http://ebook.dgbas.gov.tw/public/Data/51301351236P0LY0ZF.pdf.

Evans, D. M. Emrys. 1987. *Constancy of Purpose: An Account of the Foundation and History of the Hong Kong College of Medicine and the Faculty of Medicine of the University of Hong Kong, 1887–1987*. Hong Kong: Hong Kong University Press.

Frenk, Julio, Lincoln Chen, Zulfiqar A. Bhutta, Jordan Cohen, Nigel Crisp, Timothy Evans, Harvey Fineberg, Patricia Garcia, Yang Ke, Patrick Kelley, Barry Kistnasamy, Afaf Meleis, David Naylor, Ariel Pablos-Mendez, Srinath Reddy, Susan Scrimshaw, Jaime Sepulveda, David Serwadda, and Huda Zurayk. 2010. "Health Professionals for a New Century: Transforming Education to Strengthen Health Systems in an Interdependent World." *The Lancet* 376, no. 9756 (2010): 5–40.

Friedlander, Edward R. 2005. "Rudolf Virchow on Pathology Education." *The Pathology Guy*. Last accessed August 8, 2016. http://www.pathguy.com/virchow.htm.

General Medical Council. 2014. "Registration and Licensing." Last accessed November 11, 2015. http://www.gmc-uk.org/doctors/.

Heritage Foundation. 2014. "2014 Index of Economic Freedom." Last Accessed August 8, 2016. http://www.heritage.org/index/ranking.

Hong Kong Census and Statistics Department. 2014. "Hong Kong Annual Digest of Statistics, 2014." Last accessed August 8, 2016. http://www.censtatd.gov.hk/hkstat/sub/sp140.jsp?productCode=B1010003.

———. 2015. "National Income, Gross Domestic Product (GDP) by Economic Activity—Percentage Contribution to GDP at Basic Prices." Last accessed November 11, 2015. https://www.censtatd.gov.hk/hkstat/sub/sp250.jsp?tableID=036&ID=0&productType=8.

Kipling, Rudyard. 1889. "The Ballad of East and West." Last accessed November 11, 2015 http://www.theotherpages.org/poems/kipling01.html.

The Lancet Editors. 1892. "Conference of Medical Officers of Health." *The Lancet* 140 (3602): 621.

Licentiate Committee of the Medical Council of Hong Kong. 2014. "The 2014 Licensing Examination (Second Sitting) of the Medical Council of Hong Kong." Last Modified September 2015. http://www.mchk.org.hk/licensing_exam/index_e.htm.

Li, Choh-Ming. 1978. "Recent Developments in Medical Education." In *Chinese University Bulletin: Autumn 1978*, 16. Hong Kong: The Chinese University of Hong Kong.

Manson, Patrick. 1888. "Inaugural Address Delivered as Dean of the Hong Kong College of Medicine." *The China Review* 16: 65–73.

Matthews, Clifford N. and Oswald Cheung. 1998. *Dispersal and Renewal: Hong Kong University During the War Years*. Hong Kong: Hong Kong University Press.

National Health and Family Planning Commission of the People's Republic of China. 2013. "China Health Statistical Yearbook 2013." Last accessed November 11, 2015. http://www.nhfpc.gov.cn/htmlfiles/zwgkzt/ptjnj/year2013/index2013.html.

Organisation for Economic Co-Operation and Development. 2014. "OECD Health Statistics 2014—Frequently Requested Data." Last accessed August 8, 2016. http://www.oecd.org/els/health-systems/oecd-health-statistics-2014-frequently-requested-data.htm.

Paterson, E. H. 1987. *A Hospital for Hong Kong. The Centenary History of the Alice Ho Miu Ling Nethersole Hospital*. Hong Kong: Alice Ho Miu Ling Nethersole Hospital.

Singapore Medical Council. 2013. "Singapore Medical Council Annual Report 2013." Last accessed November 11, 2015. http://www.healthprofessionals.gov.sg/content/dam/hprof/smc/docs/annual_reports/SMC%20Annual%20Report%202013.pdf.

---. 2014. "International Medical Graduates." Last modified February 21, 2013. http://www.healthprofessionals.gov.sg/content/hprof/smc/en/leftnav/becoming_a_registereddoctor/international_medical_graduates.html.

Singapore Nursing Board. 2013. "Singapore Nursing Board Annual Report 2013." Last accessed November 11, 2015. http://www.healthprofessionals.gov.sg/content/dam/hprof/snb/docs/publications/Annual%20Report%202013.pdf.

Singapore Traditional Chinese Medicine Practitioners Board. 2012. "Singapore Traditional Chinese Medicine Practitioners Board Annual Report 2012." Last accessed November 11, 2015. http://www.healthprofessionals.gov.sg/content/dam/hprof/tcmpb/docs/Publications/TCM_AR2012.pdf.

Tao, Julia. 2006. "Confucian Care-Based Philosophical Foundation of Health Care." In *Hong Kong's Health System: Reflections, Perspectives and Visions*, edited by Gabriel M. Leung and John Bacon-Shone, 41–60.

Tsang, Steve Yui-Sang. 2004. *A Modern History of Hong Kong*. London: I. B. Tauris.

Wu, Yu-Lin. 1995. *Memories of Dr. Wu Lien-Teh, Plague Fighter*. Singapore: World Scientific.

6 The Roots of Modern Japanese Medical Education

Kenichi Ohmi

MOVING INTO AND through the twentieth century, Japan experienced dramatic political changes, from imperialism to occupation to postwar reconstruction. Its system of medical education was intertwined in these wider forces and, consequently, was radically transformed in just over 150 years. Understanding these historical influences is the key to understanding the distinctiveness of Japan's medical educational system today, so this chapter traces the course of medical education from the Edo period (1603–1867) to the present. The chapter has three main objectives: (1) to describe historical influences and paths of medical education in Japan; (2) to highlight Japanese influences on medical education in colonial Korea and Taiwan; and (3) to outline Japan's current system of medical education and examine the challenges it faces.

Historical Roots and the Meiji Restoration

In premodern Japan, as in China and ancient Rome, medical practitioners were regarded as artisans and practicing medicine was regarded as "low-grade work" (Fuse 1979, 2). For several centuries preceding the 1868 Meiji Restoration, Japanese society in the Edo period was divided roughly into four classes: samurai, which was the ruling class; followed by farmers; artisans; and merchants. These class divisions were tied to strictly ranked social status and constrained by hereditary privilege. There were very few channels through which commoners could attain upward mobility in social standing. Both study of medicine and study of Confucianism were among the exceptions, but medical practitioners were not respected as much as Confucian scholars. Medical practitioners had more material wealth but were regarded as more concerned with individuals than society, whereas Confucian scholars, while poor, were esteemed for their concern about the world more broadly (Fuse 1979). Moreover, medical practice was considered to be an artisan practice, and medical practice for payment was considered to be a merchant activity and, thus, of the lowest class.

Chinese medicine was introduced to Japan more than a thousand years ago, although it did not reach the common people until the Edo period. During the

Edo period, the Japanese practiced both Chinese medicine, referred to as *kampo* (漢方), and Western medicine, *ranpo* (蘭方), meaning Dutch medicine (also known as *Rangaku* [蘭学], meaning "Dutch Studies"). While Japanese medical practitioners accepted remedies from both medical systems in practice, they were less interested in their theoretical backgrounds, such as the yin-yang theory, the five-element theory, or the humoral theory in Western medicine. Although it was possible to practice medicine without a license or formal education during this period, there were essentially two ways to become a doctor. One way was to study medical texts under scholar-doctors or Confucian scholars. Another was to become an apprentice to a practitioner. Certification was not required in order to practice medicine, and the government did not interfere with or regulate medical practice (Fuse 1979). Although there are no statistics on medical practitioners during the Edo period, in 1876–1877, ten years after the Meiji Restoration, there were thirty thousand medical practitioners in Japan. More than ten thousand were registered as doctors of Western medicine (Aoki and Iwabuchi 2004). (Of the thirty thousand registered doctors, twenty thousand practiced Chinese, sixty-three hundred practiced Western; and thirty-seven hundred practiced both [Central Sanitary Bureau 1875–1877]).

J. C. L. Pompe van Meerdervoort, a Dutch navy surgeon who taught in Nagasaki from 1857 to 1862, observed, "There are two types of practitioners; the high status doctors known as 'shogun medical officers' and the civil practitioners who have much lower status. So the Japanese, even now, are very pleased to be educated by medical officers, and the Japanese government requests medical officers primarily" (Kamiya 1979, 16). However, there was a popular saying that "academic doctors are not good at practice," and when people got sick, they often went to nonscholar practitioners rather than to academic doctors (Fuse 1979). These nonscholar practitioners dismissed old books as dull and unproductive and often were proud that they did not read them.

From Dutch Studies to the German Model of Medicine

Western medicine had been introduced to Japan through Dutch Studies (*Rangaku*) by the late eighteenth century (Ishida 1988). *Rangaku* was diffused rapidly and widely all over Japan, beginning with the translation of textbooks such as *New Book of Anatomy* (*Kaitai shinsho*, 1774), which was translated from the Dutch *Ontleedkundige Tafelen*, which was itself a 1734 translation by Gerrit Dicten of the 1722 German anatomy book *Anatomische Tabellen* by Johan Adam Kulmus. From 1857 to 1862, the Dutch physician J. C. L. Pompe van Meerdervoort taught Western medicine at the Nagasaki Navy Medical School (*Nagasaki kaigun denshu-sho*), which was the only national medical school at that time and the only school that taught the latest Western medicine instead of assigning outdated books. A graduate of the Training College for Military Surgeons in Utrecht, he taught from a textbook and curriculum similar to those he used as a student in Utrecht. His style of teaching, similar to the approach used in Western military medical schools rather than universities, attached importance to anatomy, chemistry, physics, pharmacy, and surgery. Thus, even before the Meiji Restoration, German medicine was being introduced into Japan through the influence of Dutch medicine by doctors trained in a military style (Ishida 2007a).

Japan began to absorb Western ideas and adapt Western practices extensively during the Meiji period, and this applied to medicine as well. In 1869, the new Japanese government promptly decided to adopt a medical system based on German medicine, including its educational system (ibid.). At that time, before the medical establishment fully accepted the revolutionary knowledge that Louis Pasteur and Robert Koch were generating in their labs about bacteria, the advantage of German medicine was not obvious, so there was a broad argument in Japan about what type of medicine the country should adopt (Kamiya 1979). Sagara Tomoyasu (1836–1906), president of Tokyo Medical School (subsequently Tokyo University), reminisced that he had recommended the adoption of German medicine: "Back then Holland had influence on the world only through its translation of German or French books. Britain was arrogant and despised the Japanese, and America was too young a nation to have built up a system of medical doctors. Germany had a similar constitution as that of Japan and was a newcomer to Asia. Thus we decided to adopt German medicine" (Kamiya 1979, 10).

It seems that German medicine was adopted more for political reasons than for academic ones and that any concern for actual therapeutic efficacy possibly had even less impact on the choice than did academic concerns (Aoki 2012). In addition, there were ten thousand Western practitioners who had studied Dutch medicine in local schools or circles of *Rangaku*, and so they were more familiar with German medicine than English medicine.

Features of the German Model of Medicine

In 1871–1872, two Prussian medical officers came to Japan at the invitation of the Japanese government, and they began to reform medical education using their Prussian medical officers' school as the model. In the curriculum, all subjects were compulsory, transmission of knowledge was one-sided, importance was attached to anatomy and surgery, and there was no teaching of medical philosophy or medical history. Afterward, imperial universities and the medical professional schools that followed adopted this approach to medical education. There were several reasons why the medical officers' school model was considered suitable. First, army surgeons were regarded as having the same status as senior officials, corresponding to the warrior samurai class in Japan. Second, the top-down style of the military medical school resonated with the early Meiji period's emphasis on efficiency as a pathway to immediate modernization (Nakagawa

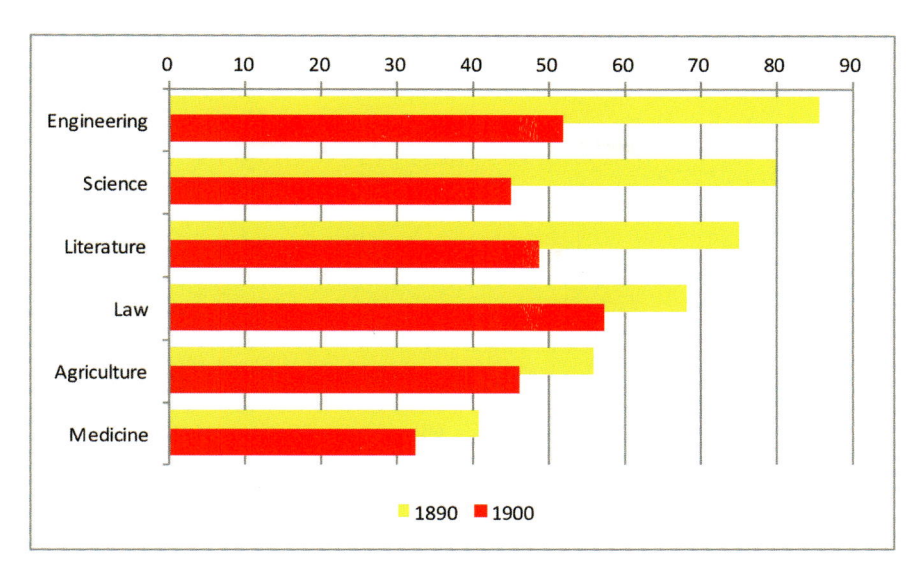

Fig. 6.1 Percentage of Descendants of Samurai at the Imperial University by Faculty.
Sources: Data from Amano 1993 and Amano 1989.

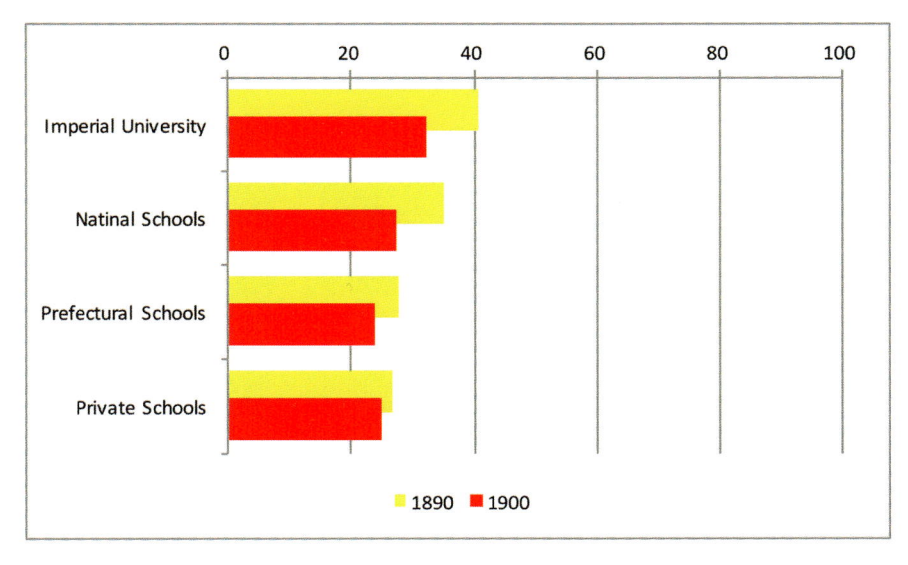

Fig. 6.2 Percentage of Descendants of Samurai at the Imperial University and Medical Professional Schools.
Sources: Data from Amano 1993 and Amano 1989.

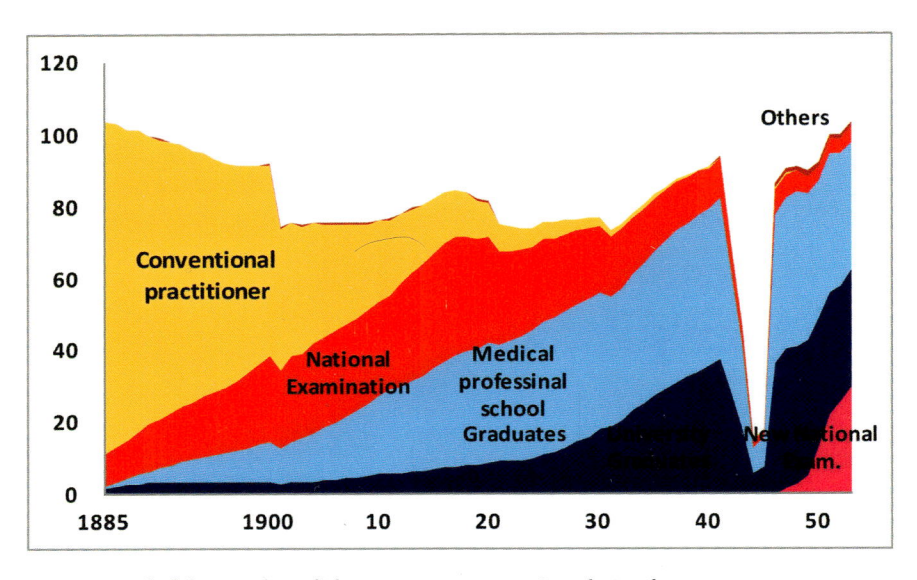

Fig. 6.3 Trend of the Number of Physicians per 100,000 Population from 1885 to 1953.
Source: Data from Bureau of Medicine, Ministry of Health and Welfare 1976.
Note: Data from before 1900 was collected from registers of physicians, and data from after 1901 was collected from surveys of physicians.

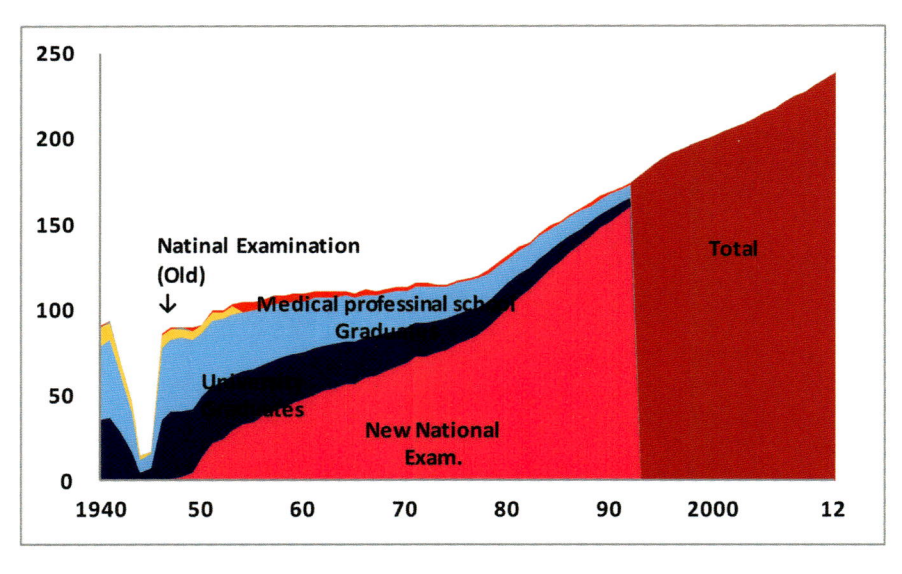

Fig. 6.4 Trends in the Number of Physicians per 100,000 Population from 1940 to 2012.
Sources: Data from Bureau of Medicine, Ministry of Health and Welfare 1976 and Statistics and Information Department, Minister's Secretariat, Ministry of Health and Welfare 1974–2012.
Note: "Certified by New National Exam" denotes physicians certified by the new 1946 National Exam only. After 1992, separate data was no longer available from licensing information.

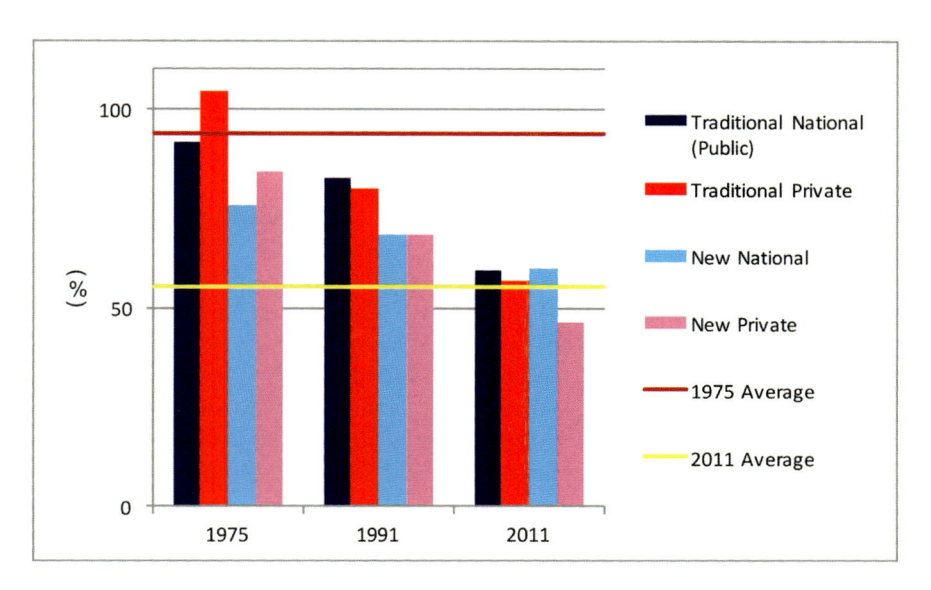

Fig. 6.5 Proportions of Numbers of Hours in the Last (Sixth) Year of Degree Program in Comparison with Averages of Those of First–Fifth Year from 1975 to 2011 by Percentage.
Source: Data from Association of Japanese Medical Colleges 1975, 1991, and 2011.

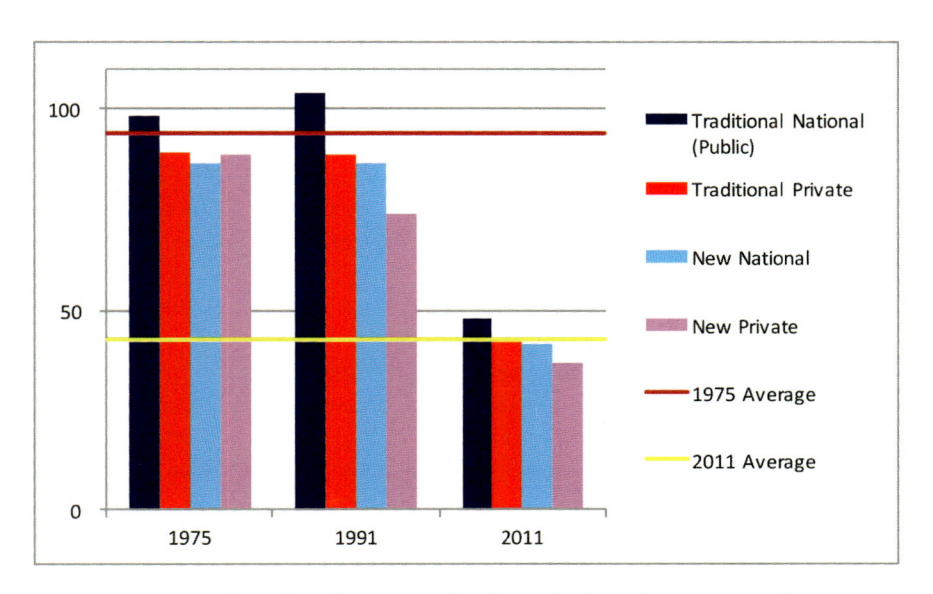

Fig. 6.6 Proportion of Number of Hours in Liberal Arts Study in Comparison with Averages of Number in Total Hours in First to Second Years of Study from 1975 to 2011 by Percentage.
Source: Data from Association of Japanese Medical Colleges 1975, 1991, and 2011.
Note: "Liberal Arts Study" includes the study of languages and sciences for medical use, often learned in the third to-fourth years of study, in addition to general "liberal arts studies" such as literature, natural sciences, history, philosophy and so on, often learned in the first to-second years of study.

1993; Kamiya 1984). Third, the Prussian medical officers' school system seemed familiar to Japanese doctors who had studied under Pompe van Meerdervoort, who was a graduate of the Training College for Military Surgeons in Utrecht and taught with similar textbooks and curriculum (Ishida 1988).

Therefore, the model of the Prussian medical officers' school, rather than that of the more common medical education system in Germany, became the foundation for the Japanese medical education system. In general, German medicine was recognized as being academic, attaching great importance to research institutes and stressing basic science and laboratory teaching, bacteriology, pathology, histology, and other such academic studies. On the other hand, the medical training taught in the Prussian medical officers' school was militaristic as well as academic. Its curriculum emphasized basic science, especially anatomy, and regarded surgery and surgical practice as being of the greatest importance (Ishida 2008).

The Japanese, however, did not adopt the Prussian medical officers' school system completely. Clinical practice and practitioners were held in low esteem, a legacy of the Edo period (Fuse 1979). The Japanese Imperial University in the late 1800s emphasized "liberal arts," and its students were required to have completed three years in higher schools or preparatory courses (after graduation from five years of junior high school) before enrollment. Higher schools corresponded to colleges and were schools for studying liberal arts, especially German language, philosophy, and literature. Consequently, the Japanese curriculum emphasized lectures, reading, and liberal arts over practical training.

Figures 6.1 and 6.2 show the percentages of descendants of samurai who attended the Imperial University and medical professional schools. Figure 6.1 shows that, in 1890, descendants of samurai were more attracted to engineering and the sciences than to literature or law. However, in 1900, descendants of samurai returned to Edo sensibilities, choosing the field of law as a substitute for Confucianism and as a path for engaging with Japanese society and the world intellectually in ways once suitable for the samurai class. The figure also shows that medicine was the least popular field of study, and the percentage of those who studied medicine decreased, most likely due to persistent ideas about class divisions, in which medical doctors were considered to be artisans.

Furthermore, Figure 6.2 shows that more descendants of samurai studied at the Imperial University than at medical professional schools and that more attended national medical professional schools than attended prefectural or private schools. In the Edo period, the public sector was identical with samurai-class work, whereas the private sector was associated with the merchant class and profit seeking and was, therefore, considered less worthy. This attitude of respecting the national and denigrating the private remained in modern Japan and was called "Kanson-Minpi [官尊民卑] [making much of officialdom and little of the people]."

Meiji-Era Reforms for Medical Practice

In 1874, shortly after the Japanese government's decision to adopt German medicine, a new Medical Law (*Isei*) was enacted under the Medical Bureau of the Ministry of Education. The Medical Law inaugurated a licensing system for practitioners, putting into place a National Examination for Medical Practitioners (Aoki 2012). The aim of the licensure system was to produce modern physicians who demonstrated their qualifications by passing a standardized examination based on knowledge of Western (i.e., German) medicine. Starting in 1876, the licensure system was controlled by the Central Sanitary Bureau of the Department for Home (domestic) Affairs (Sanitary Bureau 1925; Bureau of Medicine 1976).

The examination consisted of subjects from Western medicine, and it did not include any *kampo* medicine, a form of Chinese medicine practiced in Japan for centuries. Physicians already practicing *kampo* were considered exceptions under the new policy and permitted to continue their practice. They were known as "conventional practitioners," but after their deaths, *kampo* was no longer officially recognized.

While the national examination and licensing systems were under the jurisdiction of the Central Sanitary Bureau of the Department for Home (domestic) Affairs, imperial universities and medical professional schools were under the jurisdiction of the Department for Education (Hashimoto 1992; Hashimoto 2003b). Therefore, the Central Sanitary Bureau prioritized the number of physicians licensed to practice medicine, while the Department for Education aimed at educating high-quality physicians.

At this time, medical schools of imperial universities were situated at the top of the medical education system, and when the National Examination was introduced in 1876, graduates of imperial universities were exempt from taking it (Nakayama 1978). Graduates of Tokyo Medical School (subsequently Imperial University, or Tokyo University) obtained licenses as physicians automatically upon graduation, without examination. In general, students who entered imperial universities did so after graduating from higher schools (which corresponded to colleges in Western higher education systems), and they studied for four years, with courses mainly taught in German. In contrast, students who entered medical professional schools did so after completing junior high school, and they studied for four years, with courses mainly taught in Japanese (Amano 1993). Under this structure, medical professional schools were thought to correspond to higher schools, and were regarded as second-class schools for medical education (see Table 6.1).

At first, the privilege of obtaining a license without passing the National Examination was given only to students at medical schools of imperial universities, but in 1882, it was extended to those of other medical colleges and professional

Table 6.1. Number of Medical Schools in Japan from 1885 to 1979.

	Universities/Colleges				Medical Professional Schools		
	Imperial	National	Prefectural	Private	National	Prefectural	Private
1885	1	0	0	0	0	21	-
1888	1	0	0	0	5	3	-
1905	3	0	0	0	5	3	2
1918	4	0	1	0	5	2	5
1939	7	6	1	3	0	0	9
1945	7	6	1	4	6	18	9
	-	-	-	-	13*	1*	4*
1952	19	14	13	-	-	-	-
1969	24	9	13	-	-	-	-
1979	43	8	29	-	-	-	-

*"Provisional Medical Professional Schools" in wartime.
Source: Data from Sakai 2010.

schools. Only forty years after its establishment, the National Examination for Medical Practitioners had become a nominal exercise, and it was abolished in 1916 (Sakai 2012). Between the abolishment of the exam and the end of World War II, the way to become a licensed physician was to attend medical school (see Table 6.1).

Figure 6.3 shows the number of physicians per 100,000 population from 1885 to 1953. In 1885, the total number of physicians was approximately 40,000, making a ratio of 104 physicians per 100,000 population. More than 90 percent were conventional practitioners who had been practicing *kampo* and other traditional forms before the National Examination was introduced and who were allowed to continue doing so until they died. Over time, as the Western form of medical education took root and conventional practitioners aged or died, the percentages began to shift. In 1901, 53.8 percent of all physicians were conventional practitioners, 29 percent were physicians who had passed the National Examination, 13 percent were graduates of medical professional schools, and only 3.9 percent were graduates of imperial universities. In the 1900s and 1910s, one-third of physicians were conventional practitioners, one-third were licensed by the National Exam, and the remaining third were graduates of medical professional schools. By 1915, the number of physicians who qualified by graduating from medical professional schools reached above one-third of all physicians, and by 1929, the figure was 50 percent. Conventional practitioners, meanwhile, continued their decline, constituting only 9.7 percent of the total number of physicians in 1921 and 5.0 percent in 1927.

However, this did not translate into greater numbers of physicians. In fact, the number of new physicians of Western medicine, including those who passed the National Exam and graduates of imperial universities and medical professional schools, was insufficient and could not keep pace as the ranks of conventional practitioners began to decline. The number of physicians per 100,000 population decreased to 74.3 in 1901 due to the reduction in the number of conventional practitioners (physicians), and then it remained relatively unchanged, staying at around 80 per 100,000 population, until 1930.

The medical education system in Japan that developed under the 1873 Medical Law was a hierarchical system that classified medical schools and their graduates by rank. Imperial universities were for educating the elite, while medical professional schools were where larger numbers of physicians were educated (Hashimoto 1992). In 1885, there was one Imperial University and twenty-one prefectural medical professional schools. In 1905, there were three imperial universities, while medical professional schools had decreased to a total of ten because the central government ordered local governments to stop budgetary support to medical professional schools and many schools were closed in 1887 (see Table 6.1).

The medical professional schools, which were regarded as second-class schools, consisted of students from a wide variety of backgrounds. Many prefectural public schools, which were regarded as the educational centers of their districts and were recognized with local pride, attracted talented young students from the provinces. After the closure of medical professional schools in 1887, many schools survived as public hospitals and some of them were later restored as colleges or even as an imperial university (Sakai 2012; Shimura 2012).

However, the varied educational-degree backgrounds among physicians produced gaps in status, as shown in Table 6.2, echoing the situation found in the Edo period (Fuse 1979). In this pyramidal ordering of physicians in Japanese society and in the field of medicine in the early twentieth century, scholar-doctors were the most deeply respected. In contrast, medical practitioners were not as highly regarded, despite the fact that patients often preferred them because their clinical techniques were recognized as frequently being better than those of the scholar-doctors.

Private medical schools were long regarded in Japan as lower-class schools, even lower than prefectural public medical schools. These private medical schools attracted students from a wide variety of backgrounds, and some set themselves apart by teaching in the Anglo-American tradition. For example, Keio-gijuku Medical School (慶應義塾医学所), founded in 1873, taught medicine in the Anglo-American tradition. Although it closed in 1880, it reopened in 1916 as the School of Medicine of Keio University under Kitasato Shibasaburo (Keio University 1958; Keio University School of Medicine 1940 and 1983). In 1886, Seii-kai (成医会講習所; subsequently Jikei University) was founded by Takaki Kanehiro,

Table 6.2. Status Gap among Physicians in Japan before World War II.

High Ranking	Doctors of Medicine (graduated from imperial universities)
	Bachelors of Medicine (graduated from medical professional schools)
Between High and Middle	Degrees from foreign university or college
Middle Ranking	Graduates of the Abridged Course at Tokyo University
	Graduates of medical professional schools
Between Middle and Low	Graduates of old medical professional schools
Low Ranking	Physicians who passed the National Examination (both with or without formal study)
	Conventional practitioners (physicians)

Sources: Data from Hashimoto 2003b and Nagao 1908.

who studied medicine under William Willis (1837 1894), foreign advisor to the Japanese government, and then went to England to study at St. Thomas Hospital Medical School, which of course taught English medicine (Jikei University School of Medicine 1965; Jikei University School of Medicine 1980). Tokyo Women's Medical School (私立東京女医学校; subsequently Tokyo Women's Medical University) was founded by Yoshioka Yayoi in 1904 and was Japan's first women's medical school (Tokyo Women's Medical University 2000). Despite the quality of these institutions, there was a lingering sense inherited from the Edo period of respecting national and prefectural universities and schools and denigrating private schools (Kamiya 1984; Shimura 2012).

Simplification of the Medical Education System

The hierarchical system that existed before World War II improved the level of medical education and contributed to a more widespread diffusion of modern medicine in Japan. The system also provided medical education for more students in a relatively short time.

However, the complexity of the medical education system produced conflict between imperial universities and medical professional schools. In the 1900s, the notion of integration of the medical education system became an important issue for the Department of Education, imperial universities, and medical professional schools (Kamiya 1984). For the Ministry of Education and imperial universities, simplification meant the expansion of the imperial universities. (This process was already underway: imperial universities were built in Kyoto in 1897, in Tohoku in 1907, in Kyushu in 1911, in Hokkaido 1918, in Osaka in 1931, and in Nagoya in 1939 [Amano 2009].) On the other hand, for medical professional schools, regardless of whether they were national, prefectural, or private, simplification meant the elevation of medical professional schools to medical colleges. Most of the medical professional schools, especially the private ones, took their model from the American university and college system.

In 1918, as a compromise designed to reduce problems between the two types of schools, the government enacted the Order for Universities and Colleges (Kamiya 1984). According to this order, thirteen medical professional schools (five national, four prefectural, and four private) were elevated to the status of medical colleges (see Table 6.1). In addition, after 1939, provisional medical professional schools were established during wartime: thirteen national, one prefectural, and four private. In 1945, there were eighteen universities or medical colleges and fifty-one medical professional schools (eighteen that opened during World War II and thirty-three that opened before the war), comprising a total of sixty-nine medical schools in Japan proper (see Table 6.1 above) (Kamiya 1992; Fukushima 2012).

Japanese Influence on Medical Education in its Former Colonies

In the first half of the twentieth century, the Japanese government established a similar system for medical education in its then-colonial territories Korea and Taiwan. Graduates of imperial universities in Japan aspired to be scholar-doctors at the university level, so excellent graduates became faculty at newly established imperial universities in Korea and Taiwan (Izumi 2012). The Japanese government built both imperial universities and medical professional schools in its colonies, modeled after schools in Japan. For example, the curriculum of the medical school of Taihoku Imperial University (Taipei [台北]) was identical to that of Kyushu Imperial University, which was the Japanese university located the closest to Taiwan (Taihoku Imperial University 1936; Kyushu Imperial University 1936).

Korea Imperial University (Keijo, Seoul [京城],) was established in 1924, and Taiwan Imperial University (Taihoku, Taipei [台北],) was established in 1928 (Taihoku Imperial University 1936; Kyushu Imperial University 1936). Medical students in the Japanese colonies included Japanese, Koreans, and Taiwanese from different geographic areas and social backgrounds (Izumi 2009). In addition, medical schools were established solely for local populations and for women. For example, Severance Medical Professional School had its roots in the Medical Training Center at Jejungwong, which Horace Allen established in 1886. This private medical professional school for Koreans graduated its first class of seven students in 1908; by 1945, it had generated a thousand graduates and almost all were Korean. Additionally, Keijo Women's Medical Professional School Seoul [京城] was a private school for women (Izumi 2012; Ishida 2007).

Table 6.3 shows the estimated numbers of medical school graduates in Korea until 1945. It is estimated that the medical schools in Korea trained sixty-five

142 | *Medical Education in East Asia*

Table 6.3. Estimated Numbers of Graduates of Medical Schools in Korea until 1945.

Medical Schools	Japanese	Korean	Total
Keijo (Seoul [京城]) Imperial University	750	250	1,000
Keijo (Seoul [京城]) Medical Professional School	1,200	1,100	2,300
Severance Medical Professional School	-	1,000	1,000
Keijo (Seoul [京城]) Women's Medical Professional School	10	190	200
Heijo (Pyongyang [平壤]) Medical Professional School	600	400	1,000
Taikyuu (Daegu [大邱]) Medical Professional School	600	400	1,000
Total	3,160	3,340	6,500

Sources: Data from Ishida 2007b and Sato 1955.

hundred physicians (3,160 Japanese and 3,340 Korean). The number of Japanese graduates from Keijo Imperial University was three times as many as that of Koreans. The number of Japanese graduates from Keijo (Seoul [京城]), Heijo (Pyongyang [平壤]), and Taikyuu (Daegu [大邱]) medical professional schools was nearly equivalent to that of Korean graduates (Ishida 2007; Sato 1955). School fees at these medical schools in Japan's overseas territories were very low, or free, so that poor local people could have the opportunity to become doctors (Izumi 2009; Izumi 2012).

After World War II, medical schools in Korea continued as universities and colleges (see Table 6.4). The Japanese graduates of Japanese medical schools in Korea and Taiwan who entered before 1942 were licensed as physicians, and those who entered after 1943 were enrolled in Japanese medical schools (Izumi 2012).

Establishment of Private Medical Professional Schools and Provisional Medical Professional Schools in Wartime

Some medical professional schools and the Department of Home (domestic) Affairs in the Ministry of Army and Navy argued for the importance of producing medical practitioners rather than academic scholar-doctors and promoted the establishment of new medical professional schools (Amano 2012). By 1928, nine medical professional schools had been established (see Table 6.1). In addition, after 1939, provisional medical professional schools were set up during

Table 6.4. Medical Schools in Korea before World War II and Succeeding Schools after World War II.

Schools (Years of Establishment)	Succeeding Schools After World War II
Keijo (Seoul [京城]) Imperial University (1926)	Medical School of Seoul National University (ソウル大学校医科大学)
Keijo (Seoul [京城]) Medical Professional School (1916)	
Heijo (Pyongyang [平壌]) Medical Professional School (1933)	Pyongyang Medical College (平壌医学大学)
Taikyuu (Daegu [大邱]) Medical Professional School (1933)	Medical School of Kyungpook National University (慶北大学校医科大学)
Severance Medical Professional School (1909)	Medical School of Yonsei University (延世大学校医科大学)
Koshu (Kwangju [光州]) Medical Professional School (1943)	Medical School of Chonnam National University (全南大学校医科大学)
Kankyo (Hamgyeong [咸鏡]) Medical Professional School (1943)	Hamgyeong Medical College (咸鏡医科大学)
Keijo (Seoul [京城]) Women's Medical Professional School (1938)	Medical School of Korea University (高麗大学校医科大学)

Sources: Data from Izumi 2009 and Izumi 2012.

World War II. Thirteen national, one prefectural, and four private institutions were established (Kamiya 1992; Fukushima 2012).

Reforms after World War II: Shifting toward the American Model

The Japanese medical education system was fundamentally reformed during the post–World War II occupation by the Allied nations, known as GHQ/SCAP (General Headquarters/Supreme Commander for the Allied Powers). The reform was conducted by the Public Health and Welfare Section (PHW) of GHQ/SCAP, headed by Crawford F. Sams (1902–1994) (Kamiya 1992; Hashimoto 2003a, 2003b, and 2004). Sams entered Washington University School of Medicine in 1925, and therefore the reforms based on the 1910 Flexner Report were incorporated into his studies (Fukushima 2012). Indeed, he and the PHW reformed the Japanese medical system following the Flexner model, which consisted of: (1) reducing the number of medical schools and poorly trained physicians, (2) increasing the number of prerequisites to enter medical training, (3) training physicians to practice in a scientific manner and engage medical faculty in research, (4) giving medical schools control of clinical instruction in hospitals, and (5) regulating medical licensure (Fukushima 2012; Sugiyama 1995; Sams 1986). Sams created the Council on Medical Education (CME) in Japan, whose objective was to restructure Japanese medical education and to eliminate inadequate medical schools. He appointed Kusama Yoshio (草間良男) (1888–1968), who was professor of hygiene at Keio University and who had studied at Stanford University and Johns Hopkins University School of Medicine, as chairman of the committee (Hashimoto 2008).

Elimination and Consolidation of Medical Professional Schools

As mentioned earlier, in 1945 there were eighteen universities or medical colleges and fifty-one medical professional schools in Japan (see Table 6.1). CME conducted a survey of medical professional schools and subsequently classified them into twenty-one "A class" schools and twenty-four "B class" schools, with the latter judged to be providing inadequate instruction. The "B class" schools were closed, following the principles of the Flexner reform (Fukushima 2012). In 1952, Japan's medical schools were reorganized into forty-six universities and colleges (nineteen national, fourteen prefectural, and thirteen private) (Nakagawa 1988).

Changes in Courses and Curriculums

The courses at the medical schools of universities and colleges and at medical professional schools were unified and modified into a seven-year curriculum: two years of liberal arts, two years of basic sciences, and two years of clinical medicine, followed by a one-year internship at a teaching hospital. Before World War II, almost 70 percent of the curriculums in medical schools was devoted to lectures, and the remaining 30 percent was for experiments and clinical training, including "clinical lectures," in which patients were taken into large lecture halls. In 1947, the Japan University Accreditation Association (JUAA), a voluntary organization of higher education institutions, was established using several US accreditation agencies as a model. In 1948, the JUAA adopted a unified standard for medical education. It required that clinical training make up 53 percent of the curriculum and specified strict percentages for other subjects: 10 percent for anatomy; 19 percent for internal medicine; and 9 percent for surgery. It prioritized social medicine (2 percent for hygiene and 4 percent for public health) and clinical medicine over basic sciences and internal medicine over surgery (Fukushima 2012; Sugiyama 1995).

Before World War II, graduates of universities and medical colleges often practiced without clinical training. For clinical training, a postgraduate one-year internship was introduced into the Japanese medical education system, following the model of Flexner reforms. However, Sams was anxious about this internship system because interns were nonsalaried and they were already overworked in preparing for the National Examination (Fukushima 2012; Sugiyama 1995).

National Examination for Physicians

In 1916, the National Examination for Medical Practitioners was abolished and all graduates—whether from imperial universities, public medical professional schools, or private medical professional schools—received qualification as physicians upon graduation (Hashimoto 2003b). In the autumn of 1946, a new National Examination for Physicians was introduced and all new graduates of medical schools were required to pass this examination in order to be certified as physicians (Fukushima 2012).

Figure 6.4 shows that the numbers and percentages of physicians certified through this new examination system increased steadily. In 1950, only 14 percent of all physicians had passed the exam, followed by 33 percent in 1955, 44 percent in 1960, 60 percent in 1970, and 77 percent in 1980. Finally, in 1992, the last year that data from licensing information was available, 92 percent of graduates had passed the examination.

Great Changes in Society and Minor Changes in Medical Education in the 1950s and 1960s

In the postwar period, Japan experienced great demographic changes and health transitions. Mortality patterns in Japan shifted from high mortality in youth, primarily due to infectious diseases, to low mortality overall, with the majority being elderly persons passing away due to chronic diseases. In 1935–1936, life expectancy in Japan was forty-seven years for males and fifty for females. In 1947, life expectancy increased to fifty years for males and fifty-four for females, and by 1960 it had reached sixty-five for males and seventy for females (Health, Labour, and Welfare Statistics Association 2010).

After World War II, there seemed to be too many physicians, including a large number of graduates from medical schools and from provisional medical professional schools established during the war (Kamiya 1992). Nonetheless, this seemingly excessive number of physicians, in part, enabled Japan to achieve a universal health insurance system, which was realized in 1961. Before the war, a Health Insurance Law was established in 1927 for workers in factories and mines, but it covered only 2 million (3.3 percent) Japanese. In 1938, the National Health Insurance Law expanded coverage to rural areas and to small business employees, reaching a total of 6.7 million people (9.3 percent). The increased number of physicians, combined with rapid economic growth, enabled Japan to introduce the New National Health Insurance system in 1958 and achieve universal health insurance coverage in 1961 (Hashimoto 1996).

After 1961, the number of patients per physician continued to increase. The number of patients per physician was twenty-seven in 1955, and it rose to thirty-six in 1960, forty-four in 1965, and fifty-one in 1969. The number of medical schools remained almost unchanged until 1970, after which it increased (Hashimoto 1996).

In the 1950s and 1960s, the Japanese government modified only the medical curriculum. The internship system was not changed to a clinical training system until 1968 (Fukushima 2012). That year marked the start of the actual implementation of the clinical training system instead of the intern system. After that, clinical training was done after passing the National Examination. Thus, these trainees came to their clinical training as "doctors," freed from concerns about salaries and passing the National Exam, and patients received care from "doctors" instead of "students."

1970s and After: Diffusion of the American Model

In the 1970s, many medical schools were established in Japan and the number of medical schools, which had remained unchanged from 1955 to 1970 at forty-six, increased to eighty. Most of the new medical schools were separate colleges, rather than departments of universities, and it was hoped that they would lead to innovations in medical education, accelerating the reforms of the 1950s and 1960s toward implementing medicine based on the American model (Hashimoto 2008).

The Standards for Establishing Medical Schools written in 1968, just before the surge of new medical schools, aimed to make the curriculum of every school independent and reduce the restrictions placed on them, such as the JUAA unified standard requirement mentioned above (Fukushima 2012). Among the newly established medical schools, eighteen national schools were situated in smaller cities, and sixteen private schools, all of which belonged to educational foundations, were located in Tokyo or other large cities (Hashimoto 2008). An unintended consequence of the 1946 reimplementation of the National Examination for Physicians, a postwar reform based on the American model of medical education, was that the newly established medical schools adopted cramming-oriented curriculums. This was done in order to raise their exam pass rates and thereby attract students, most of whom were the children of medical practitioners. Graduates of older schools, especially those of national public schools, looked down on the graduates of these new schools, whom they regarded as "crammers," just as previous generations of elites had done before to the practitioners who took the National Examination for medical licensing. And so, ironically, despite the fact that after the war all doctors had to pass the National Exam in order to practice medicine, there was still a tendency to look down on those who graduated from the new private medical schools.

Figure 6.4 shows that the number of physicians per 100,000 population remained unchanged at slightly above 100 from 1954 until 1980. After the establishment of the new medical schools, the number of physicians increased rapidly and went over 150 per 100,000 population in 1986 and over 200 in 2000, reaching 238 in 2012. Newly established schools contributed to a more equal distribution of physicians across Japan's prefectures, but they also contributed to a growing disparity in the distribution of physicians within each prefecture because they often decided to work or practice in prefectural capital cities, rather than in rural areas (Toyokawa et al. 2007).

The Present State of the Japanese Medical Education System

Types of Medical Schools in Japan

Japanese medical schools consist of the older national public schools that were established before 1950 and the newer national public schools that were established from 1970 to 1978 (Hashimoto 2008). The older national public schools, including former imperial universities and national medical professional schools, acted as centers of medicine and medical education in several areas of Japan and fostered the teaching staffs of medical schools.

Traditional private schools, which developed from private medical professional schools, enrolled students from a wide variety of backgrounds but were generally regarded as second-class schools. Some private schools taught Anglo-American medicine, including a women's medical school. In local areas, private medical professional schools were established as alternatives to prefectural public schools, with assistance from local volunteers, and each one was recognized with local pride as being "our school." However, private schools have never been considered to be as elite as public schools.

Newer national public schools were established in local areas that were short of physicians, in accordance with the policy that every prefecture should have at least one medical school. An exception was the University of Tsukuba, established in 1973, which was established as a model of the new medical education system that focused on education and training for students rather than faculty research and created curriculums that integrated basic science, clinical lectures, and training. New private schools were established in urban areas in order to produce more physicians because most practitioners were located in urban areas and wanted to see their children become physicians and eventually take over their clinics.

Recent Changes in the Japanese Medical Education System

Table 6.5 shows changes at medical schools from 1975 to 2011. In 1975, the average total number of hours in the curriculums of all eighty medical schools designated for medical education, including lectures, experiments, bedside training, and other associated training, was 6,312. This number decreased by about 1,000 hours to 5,337 hours in 2011. Dividing medical education into (1) liberal arts, (2) clinical lectures, and (3) clinical training, we can see that, from 1975 to 2011, the

Table 6.5. Changes at Medical Schools from 1975 to 2011.

Average Number of Hours of Medical Education

	Traditional		New		(Former Imperial)	Total
	National (Public)	Private	National (Public)	Private		
1975	6,150	6,712	6,137	6,380	(5,903)	6,312
1991	5,832	6,025	5,709	5,736	(6,281)	5,803
2011	5,200	5,313	5,611	5,236	(5,333)	5,337

Average Number of Hours of Liberal Arts in Medical Education

	Traditional		New		(Former Imperial)	Total
	National (Public)	Private	National (Public)	Private		
1975	1,608	1,945	1,761	1,767	(1,616)	1,716
1991	1,732	1,577	1,568	1,412	(2,132)	1,591
2011	762	723	687	677	(1,066)	714

Average Number of Hours of Clinical Lectures in Medical Education

	Traditional		New		(Former Imperial)	Total
	National (Public)	Private	National (Public)	Private		
1975	2,717	2,766	3,055	2,799	(2,477)	2,757
1991	2,402	2,402	2,254	2,574	(2,342)	2,404
2011	1,753	1,748	1,929	2,389	(1,657)	1,923

Average Number of Hours of Clinical Training in Medical Education

	Traditional		New		(Former Imperial)	Total
	National (Public)	Private	National (Public)	Private		
1975	1,794	1,899	1,208	1,721	(1,724)	1,779
1991	1,732	2,045	1,886	1,856	(1,743)	1,842
2011	2,733	2,823	2,973	2,228	(2,759)	2,727

Average Number of Hours of Medical Education in the Last Year of Degree Program (6th Year)

	Traditional		New		(Former Imperial)	Total
	National (Public)	Private	National (Public)	Private		
1975	957	1,163	809	924	(873)	997
1991	828	836	688	691	(831)	768
2011	549	544	602	447	(583)	532

Source: Data from Association of Japanese Medical Colleges 1975, 1991, and 2011.

number of hours spent in liberal arts decreased by more than 1,000, from 1,716 to 608. Similarly, the number of hours spent in clinical lectures decreased by nearly 1,000, from 2,757 to 1,923. Conversely, the number of hours spent in clinical training increased by nearly 1,000, from 1,779 to 2,727. The overall decrease of hours required for a medical education was due to the decrease in hours for liberal arts study, while the hours for clinical education (sum total of lectures and training) remained unchanged or slightly increased.

Most of the older national schools, especially the former imperial universities, resisted change more than other schools. They adhered to the principles of German medicine, prioritizing lectures and reading over clinical practice. As mentioned above, the teaching of liberal arts at medical schools in Japan has declined dramatically, although it has been better preserved at traditional schools, especially at the former imperial universities. The average number of hours devoted to liberal arts studies in 2011 was 621 at the older national (public) schools, 630 at older private schools, and 724 at former imperial universities.

Unexpectedly, from 1975 to 2011, the number of hours spent in the last year of medical degree programs (the sixth year) decreased. The average number of hours in the sixth year in all medical schools was 997 in 1975, and it decreased nearly by half, to 532, in 2011. Figure 6.5 shows the changes from 1975 to 2011, showing the proportion of hours spent in the sixth year of medical degree programs in comparison with the averages of hours spent during the first to fifth years. In particular, we can see that traditional private schools, whose bar was over 100 percent in 1975, laid stress on clinical training in hospitals, often done in the sixth year of study. The proportion decreased nearly by half, from 94 percent in 1975 to 56 percent in 2011. In other words, in 2011, students in the last year of Japanese medical degree programs studied or trained for only half the amount of time that students in their first to fifth years did. At present, the six-year medical educational system in Japan has become a world of "five and a half years" of education. Although the date for taking the National Examination was moved up from March to February in 2005, we are not able to confirm whether or not this shift in date precipitated the decreased number of hours in the sixth year.

Furthermore, Figure 6.6 shows the changes from 1975 to 2011 in the number of hours of liberal arts study in comparison with the average total number of hours of first-to-second year study. We can also see that traditional national schools (whose bars were over 100 percent in 1975 and 1991) laid stress on the liberal arts in the first-to-second years of study and on further study of languages and sciences for medical use as preparation for medical study in the third-to-fourth years of study until 1991, when the JUAA unified standard for medical education was eased significantly. The proportion decreased by more than half, from 94 percent in 1975 to 43 percent in 2011. In many medical schools, especially in relatively new private schools, the overall curriculum has been compressed and shortened, probably for the purpose of allowing students more time to study for the National Examination.

Discussion about the Future

Desired Types of Physicians in Japan before and after the War: Models, Realities, and Roots

As mentioned above, many Japanese physicians desired to be "scholar-doctors," in the Edo-period tradition of Confucian doctors. These persistent attitudes stemmed from Japan's cultural history, despite the influence of the German model of medical education in Japan. In contrast, clinical practice and experimental medicine were very important in the Prussian Medical Officers' School. In German universities, liberal arts and medical studies were well respected. Japanese medical students who studied at old Japanese higher schools and in Germany thought they were following the German model, although they did not fully grasp the importance of medical practice and experimental medicine in Germany (see Table 6.6).

The scholar-doctor tradition in prewar Japan had proved adept at producing a capable teaching staff. It is notable that excellent graduates from the scholar-doctor tradition became faculty members at newly established imperial universities, including those in Korea and Taiwan. And even the notorious "academic chair system"—in which one professor had complete control over the personnel of a department—had the merit of being able to send doctors to villages that previously had none, in accordance with a professor's order.

However, after the war, Japanese physicians began to place increasing importance on clinical training and practice over liberal arts and lectures—in marked contrast to their attitude before the war. This type of hands-on practical training had a cultural precedent in Japan with the nonscholar medical practitioners of the Edo period. Since World War II, the Japanese medical education system

Table 6.6. Desired Types of Physician in Japan before World War II (Author's Estimation).

		Liberal Arts	Clinical Lecture	Clinical Training	Experimental Medicine	Medical Research	Practitioner
Model	"German Model"	±	+	+	+	+	±
Reality	"Scholar Doctors"	+	+	−	−	+	−
Roots	"Confucian Doctors"	+	+	−	−	−	−

+: Respected ±: Neutral −: Looked down on.

Table 6.7. Desired Types of Physicians in Japan after World War II (Author's Estimation).

		Liberal Arts	Clinical Lecture	Clinical Training	Experimental Medicine	Medical Research	Practitioner
Model	"American Model"	+	+	+	+	+	+
Reality	"Practitioner Doctors"	–	–	+	±	±	+
Roots	"Non-scholar Practitioner"	–	–	+	–	–	+

+: Respected ±: Neutral –: Looked down on.

has educated physicians in the vein of nonscholar medical practitioners, placing importance on clinical training and practice, according to the principles of the American model of medical education.

An improved attitude toward medical practitioners after the war was also influenced by the adoption of the national licensing system, which resulted in the decline of the hierarchy of medical education institutions. By the 1990s, the percentage of physicians who passed the new examination exceeded 90 percent. However, one weakness has been that excessive stress has been placed on passing the National Examination at the expense of liberal arts and lectures. In the American Flexnerian system, described in depth in chapter 2, in addition to clinical training and practice, liberal arts, lectures, medical research, and experimental medicine were also highly respected, but these elements now have reduced importance at many Japanese medical schools (see Table 6.7).

Current Problems Concerning Medical Professionals in Japan

At present, the three major challenges to Japanese medical education are quantity, quality, and placement of physicians in meeting the demands placed on Japan's health care system, including the steady increase in Japan's elderly population. The Ministry of Health, Labour and Welfare and the Ministry of Education, along with medical schools and associations, have been cooperating in efforts to resolve these problems. While there is a surplus of doctors, many are reluctant to work in rural areas and the present system of postgraduate clinical programs has not been sufficient in attracting young doctors to work in unpopular rural areas. In the past, orders from the all-powerful professors or department chairmen were sufficient to deal with this problem, but today, other financial and organizational incentives are becoming necessary. This situation suggests that there has not been enough attention paid to the quality, temperament, and change in the desired types of doctors in Japan.

Following the American model of medical education, the Japanese system is now strong in clinical training and practice. Nonetheless, this system has been accompanied by an emphasis on passing the National Examination, while lectures and liberal arts education have suffered. In Japan, when a student who has graduated from medical school does not pass the National Examination, he or she will not become a doctor and will also be regarded as a dropout—a kind of "failure." When a person becomes a medical student, there is no way to receive social acceptance other than by becoming a doctor. Thus, for medical school students, passing the National Examination is an absolute must and, in selecting a medical school, students are highly influenced by the school's examination pass rate. Schools are at risk of falling into a vicious cycle: if a medical school's pass rate is lower than that of other schools, it is less able to attract excellent students and its pass ratio falls further. Consequently, medical school students are willing to do almost anything to pass the National Examination and medical schools are willing to do almost anything to raise or maintain their pass rates.

Dr. Erwin von Belz (1849–1913), a famous teacher and doctor from Germany during the Meiji era, said in his memorial lecture at the University of Tokyo that the Japanese aspired to obtain only the fruits of education, without engaging in intellectual fighting in basic fields. The results of the immediately prior section in this chapter show that, in the past twenty years, many medical schools have emphasized intensive cramming rather than steady study in order to raise or maintain their pass rates. The 2001 reform of the National Examination system seems to have accelerated the trend toward cramming: it increased the number of questions from 320 to 500 and determined that examinees pass on the basis of their score ranking, instead of on the basis of their absolute level of achievement (Japanese Society for Medical Education 2014).

It should be noted that the compression of curriculum in order to allow time for cramming begins early for Japanese students; it is a common technique employed by preparatory high schools to raise their pass rates for acceptances into prestigious universities. Considering this condition, the inattentive attitude toward the liberal arts and the stress put on passing the National Examination represent two sides of the same coin.

Furthermore, new private medical schools have particularly been affected by such problems. Formerly, it was an open secret that some new private schools practiced compressed curriculums, named the "wedged curriculum," in order to allow more time for cramming for the National Examination, but this was thought to be the case in only a very small fraction of medical schools (Hosaka 1987). However, exam pressures outlined in the previous section suggest that such weaknesses have been common in all medical schools, both old and new, national and private, for the last two decades. And as this study suggests, these challenges are rooted in Japan's cultural history and in the context in which Western models were adopted.

Many who are concerned about medical education in Japan seem to consider the emphasis on clinical practice, the inattentive attitude toward lectures and the liberal arts, and the stress put on passing the National Examination to be an intractable situation. However, this attitude relegates lectures and liberal arts courses to a lesser status, to be taught by part-time instructors, which in turn results in making these classes more dull and prosaic. Even those who formulate the questions for the National Examination often have biased attitudes, including regarding the exam as a necessary evil, and they can easily turn medical candidates into crammers. In turn, the questions on the National Exam are becoming more and more cumbersome. This leads to questions about the quality of the doctors produced by the medical education system.

In considering this situation we might heed the words of Confucius (孔子) who said, "To study and not think is a waste. To think and not study is dangerous." In thinking about the situation of medical education in Japan today, we might revise this slightly to say, "To study and not practice is a waste. To practice and not study is dangerous."

Conclusion: Moving Toward the Future

During the Edo period, Japan assimilated Western medicine. In the twentieth century, it adopted the American model of medical education and modernized the Japanese medical system. However, the present Japanese medical education system seems more similar to the "nonscholar practitioner" model rooted in the Edo period than to the American model. Accordingly, current views of medical education in Japan suggest that lectures and the liberal arts are largely useless and that cramming for the National Exam is a necessary evil. Both of these views are erroneously taken by most Japanese medical educators to have originated from the American model.

Medical educators are making efforts to reform and improve Japan's medical education system, including increasing the amount of clinical training (Japan Society for Medical Education 2014). However, there is a need to address more fundamental problems, such as limited training in the liberal arts and the overemphasis on the National Examination. As a first step toward improving Japan's current system, we should recognize and understand this background.

To improve the quality of medical education and the type of doctors Japan produces, liberal arts—including history, ethics, and behavioral sciences—should be stressed within the curriculum as a requisite part of medical study and training. In particular, the Core Curriculum in Medical Education, produced by the Research Collaborators' Conference on Improvement and Enhancement of Medical Education, should include guidelines about the liberal arts training (ibid.). Furthermore, medical colleges that are comprised of only medical schools or a few additional medically oriented faculties such as dentistry and nursing, where liberal arts are taught by part-time instructors, should enhance their teaching staffs by taking measures such as merging with or cooperating with other colleges and universities that offer such courses.

Finally, the fundamental problem of overemphasis on passing the National Examination should be addressed. In 2001, the National Examination system was reformed in an unsatisfactory direction, leading to more competition among students and among medical schools. Japan needs to re-reform the National Examination system, thereby permitting it to examine the absolute level of achievement of each student, rather than just providing a relative evaluation. This could be assisted by developing a system of evaluating examinees at various stages during their study, instead of relying only on a one-time, enormous paper test, which encourages cramming.

To solve this fundamental problem, Japan could reform certain medical schools and turn them into graduate schools, which would provide a model for the coexistence of study and practice. This proposal has two merits. First, because Japanese university or college graduates are not beholden to the same "dropout" status as medical students who do not pass the national examination, a new system could mean that students of reformed graduate medical schools who study medicine could have choices aside from becoming doctors, including research or nonmedical business. Second, this system would not allow medical schools to compress their liberal arts curriculums in order to produce time for cramming. Under such a proposed system, medical schools (graduate schools) would be able to educate well-cultured and experienced students who have a clear sense of purpose.

In order to realize these reforms, Japanese medical educators should become aware that Japan has been pursuing the wrong strategy and is heading in the wrong direction. In order to more successfully move forward in the future, Japan needs to follow another quotation from Confucius (孔子): "He that would know what shall be must consider what has been."

References

Amano, Ikuo [天野郁夫]. 1989. 近代日本高等教育研究 [*Study of Higher Education in Modern Japan*]. Tokyo: Tamagawa University Publications.
———. 1993. 旧制専門学校論 [*Study of Old Professional Schools*]. Tokyo: Tamagawa University Publications.
———. 2009. 大学の誕生 [*The Birth of the University*]. Tokyo: Chuo-koron-shinsha.
———. 2012. 大学令と大正昭和期の医師養成. 坂井建雄編 [*The University Ordinance and Training of Doctors in Taisho-Showa Period*]. In *History of Medical Education in Japan*, edited by Tatsuo Sakai, 149–85. Sendai: Tohoku University Press.
Aoki, Toshiyuki [青木歳幸]. 2012. 江戸時代の医学, 名医たちの三〇〇年 [*Medicine in Edo period: 300 Years of Excellent Physicians*]. Tokyo: Yoshikawa-kobunkan.

Aoki, Toshiyuki, Naoko Osada, and Kentaro Hosono [青木歳幸，長田直子，細野健太郎]. 2004. "地域蘭学者門人帳データベースについて [Database on Student Records of Regional Rangaku Schools]." In 青木歳幸. 共同研究　地域蘭学の総合的研究 [Collaborative Research: Comprehensive Study of Regional Rangaku: Western Sciences Study in the Edo Era Using Dutch Language Materials], edited by Toshiyuki Aoki and Reiji Iwabuchi, 国立歴史民俗学博物館研究報告 [Bulletin of the National Museum of Japanese History], vol.116: 479-95. 佐倉: 財団法人歴史民俗学博物館振興会　2004. Sakura: Foundation for Museums of Japanese History.

Association of Japanese Medical Colleges [全国医学部長病院長会議]. 1975. 医学教育カリキュラムの現状. 昭和50年, 1975 [Current Situation of Curriculums of Japanese Medical Colleges, 1975]. Tokyo: Association of Japanese Medical Colleges.

———. 1991. 医学教育カリキュラムの現状. 平成3年, 1991] [Current Situation of Curriculums of Japanese Medical Colleges, 1991]. Tokyo: Association of Japanese Medical Colleges.

———. 2011. 医学教育カリキュラムの現状. 平成23年, 2011. [Current Situation of Curriculums of Japanese Medical Colleges, 2013]. Tokyo: Association of Japanese Medical Colleges.

Bureau of Medicine, Ministry of Health and Welfare [厚生省医務局]. 1976. 医制百年史 [100 Years' History of Medical System]. Tokyo: Bureau of Medicine and Ministry of Health and Welfare.

Central Sanitary Bureau of the Department for Home Affairs [内務省衛生局]. 1875-1877. 衛生局第一第二報告, 明治8年〜10年 [First - Second Report of the Central Sanitary Bureau of the Department for Home Affairs]. Tokyo: Bureau of Medicine and Ministry of Health and Welfare.

Fukushima, Osamu [福島統]. 2012. "戦後における医学教育制度改革. 坂井建雄編. [Medical Education Reform in Post-War Period]." In History of Medical Education in Japan, edited by Tatsuo Sakai, 213-45. Sendai: Tohoku University Press.

Fuse, Shoichi (布施昌一). 1979. 医師の歴史　その日本的特徴 [History of Physicians: Japanese Features]. Tokyo: Chuou-koron-sha.

Hashimoto, Koichi [橋本鉱市]. 1992. "近代日本における専門職と資格試験制度—医術開業試験を中心として [Profession and Qualification Examination System in Modern Japan: Focusing on the National Examination for Medical Practitioners]." 教育社会学研究 [Sociology of Education] 51: 136-53.

———. 1996. "戦後日本における専門職養成政策の政治プロセス—医師を中心として [Political Process on the Plan of Educating Professionals in Post-War Japan: Focusing on the Medical Doctors]."東京大学大学院教育学研究科紀要 [University of Tokyo Graduate School of Education Bulletin] 36:41-60.

———. 2003a. "GHQ SCAP PHWと「医学教育審議会」(1)占領期医学教育改革の審議内容と政策過程, 東北大学大学院教育学研究科研究年報 [GHQ/SCAP/PHW and the Council on Medical Education: Part I: Policy-making Process of Medical Education Reform during the Occupation Period]." Tohoku University Graduate School of Education Research Annual Report 51: 29-52.

———. 2003b. "医師の「量」と「質」をめぐる政治過程. 望田幸男, 田村栄子編. 身体と医療の教育社会史 [Political Process over 'Quantity' and 'Quality' of Physicians]." In Social History of Education in Body and Medicine, edited by Y. Mochida and E. Tamura, 111-35. Kyoto: Showa-do.

———. 2004. "GHQ SCAP PHWと「医学教育審議会」(2)占領期における医学教育改革の審議内容と政策過程 [GHQ/SCAP/PHW and the Council on Medical Education: Part II: Policy-making Process of Medical Education Reform During the Occupation Period]" Tohoku University Graduate School of Education Research Annual Report 52: 63-85.

———. 2008. 専門職養成の政策過程－戦後日本の医師数をめぐって－ [*The Policy Process of Professional Training: Concerning the Number of Doctors in Japan after World War II*]. Tokyo: Gakujutu-shuppankai.
Health, Labour, and Welfare Statistics Association. 2011. 国民衛生の動向2010/2011 [*Trends in Public Health of Japan 2010-2011*]. Tokyo: Health, Labour, and Welfare Statistics Association. 2011.
Hosaka, Masayasu [保阪正康]. 1987. 大学医学部 [*Medical Schools*]. Tokyo: Kodansha.
Ishida, Sumio [石田純郎]. 1988. 蘭学の背景.思文閣出版 [*Backgrounds of Dutch Studies*]. Kyoto: Shibunkaku-shuppan.
———. 2007a. オランダにおける蘭学医書の形成.思文閣出版 [*Formation of Dutch Studies Medical Book in the Netherlands*]. Kyoto: Shibunkaku-shuppan.
———. 2007b. 韓国近代医学教育史(1876-1953) [*History of Modern Medical Education in Korea, 1876-1953*]. 一朝鮮の開国から朝鮮動乱まで、日韓併合時代を中心に. 人文科学論叢 [*The Journal of Niimi Academy of Science and Culture*] 4-5: 1-49.
Izumi, Takateru [泉孝英]. 2009. 外地の医学校 [*Medical Schools of Overseas Territories*]. Osaka: Medical Review.
———. 2012. "泉孝英. 戦時下における外地の医学校. 坂井建雄編. 日本医学教育史 [*Medical Schools of Overseas Territories in Wartime*]." In *History of Medical Education in Japan*, edited by Tatsuo Sakai, 187–211. Sendai: Tohoku University Press.
Japan Society for Medical Education [日本医学教育学会]. 2014. 医学教育白書 2014 年版 [*White Paper on Medical Education 2014*]. Tokyo: Shinohara-shuppan-shinsha.
Jikei University School of Medicine. [東京慈恵会医科大学]. 1965. 東京慈恵会医科大学八十五年史 [*Eighty-five-year History of The Jikei University School of Medicine*]. Tokyo: Jikei University School of Medicine.
———. 1980. 東京慈恵会医科大学八十五年史 [*One Hundred Year History of The Jikei University School of Medicine*]. Tokyo: Jikei University School of Medicine.
Kamiya, Akinori [神谷昭典]. 1979. 日本近代医学のあけぼの [*Emergence of Modern Medicine in Japan*]. Tokyo: Iryo-tosho-shuppan-sha.
———. 1984. 神谷昭典. 日本近代医学の定立 [*Establishment of Modern Medicine in Japan*]. Tokyo: Iryo-tosho-shuppan-sha.
———. 1992. 神谷昭典. 日本近代医学の相克 [*Conflict of Modern Medicine in Japan*]. Tokyo: Iryo-tosho-shuppan-sha.
Keio University [慶応義塾]. 1958. 慶応義塾百年史 上・中・下巻 別巻 [*Keio Hundred Years' History*]. Tokyo: Keio University.
Keio University School of Medicine [慶応義塾大学医学部]. 1940. 慶応義塾大学医学部20周年記念誌 [*Twentieth Anniversary of Keio University School of Medicine*]. Tokyo: Keio University School of Medicine.
———. 1983. 慶応義塾大学医学部60周年記念誌 [*Sixtieth Anniversary of Keio University School of Medicine*]. Tokyo: Keio University School of Medicine.
Kyushu Imperial University. 1936. 九州帝国大学一覧 昭和11年 [*The Kyushu Imperial University Calendar*]. 1936. Fukuoka: Kyushu Imperial University.
Nagao, Setsuzo [長尾折三]. 1908. 噫 医弊 [*Oh Evil in Medicine*]. Tokyo: Toho-do.
Nakagawa, Yonezo [中川米造]. 1964. 医学の弁明 [*Apology of Medicine*]. Tokyo: Seishin Shobo.
———. 1987-1988. "Adoption of Western Medicine in Japan." *Clio Medica*. 21 (1–4): 113–118.
———. 1988. 中川米造.医療の文明史 [*History of Civilization in Medicine*]. Tokyo: Japan Broadcasting Publishers Association.
———. 1993. 素顔の医者 [*Doctors Barefaced*]. Tokyo: Kodan-sha.

Nakayama, Shigeru [中山茂]. 1978. 中山茂.帝国大学の誕生 国際比較の中での東大 [Birth of Imperial University: University of Tokyo in International Comparison]. 東京 [Tokyo]: 中央公論社 [Chuo-koron-shinsha].

Sakai, Tatsuo [坂井建雄他]. 2010. "我が国の医学教育・医師資格付与制度の歴史的変遷と医学校の発展過程 [Historical Development of the Systems of Medical Education and Medical Licensure and Its Effect on Evolution of Medical Schools in Japan]." 医学教育 [Medical Education] 41 (5): 337–46.

———. 2012. "坂井建雄. 明治期初期の公立医学校. 坂井建雄編. 日本医学教育史 [Public Medical Schools of Early Meiji Period]." In History of Medical Education in Japan, edited by Tatsuo Sakia, 61–113. Sendai: Tohoku University Press.

Sams, C. F. [サムス, C. F.]. 1986. ＤＤＴ革命―占領期の医療福祉政策を回想する [DDT Revolution: Recalls of the Medical Welfare Policy of Occupation in Japan]. Tokyo: Iwanami Shoten.

Sanitary Bureau of the Department for Home Affairs [内務省衛生局]. 1925. 医制五十年史 [50 Years' History of Medical System]. 1925. Tokyo: Sanitary Bureau of the Department for Home Affairs.

Sato, Gozo [佐藤剛蔵]. 1955. "朝鮮医育史補遺 [Korea History of Medical Education: Addendum]." 朝鮮学報 [Korea Science Report] 7: 161–72.

Shimura, Toshiro [志村俊郎]. 2012. "明治期における私立医学校の教育. 坂井建雄編. 日本医学教育史 [Education in Private Medical Schools of Meiji Period]." In History of Medical Education in Japan, edited by Tatsuo Sakai, 115–47. Sendai: Tohoku University Press.

Statistics and Information Department, Minister's Secretariat, Ministry of Health and Welfare [厚生省大臣官房統計情報部]. 1974–2012. "医師・歯科医師・薬剤師調査 (1974–2012分) [Survey of Physician, Dentist, Pharmacist, 1974–2012]." Tokyo: Statistics and Information Department.

Sugiyama, Akiko. [杉山章子]. 1995. 占領期の医療改革 [Healthcare Reform in Occupation Period]. Tokyo: Keiso-shobo.

Taihoku Imperial University. 1936. 台北帝国大学一覧 昭和11年 [The Taihoku Imperial University Calendar]. Taipei: Taihoku Imperial University.

Terumi, Mikami [三上昭美]. 1966. 東京女子医科大学小史 [Brief History of Tokyo Women's Medical University]. Tokyo: Tokyo Women's Medical University.

Tokyo Women's Medical University [東京女子医科大学]. 2000. 東京女子医科大学百年史 [Tokyo Women's Medical University Hundred Year History]. Tokyo: Tokyo Women's Medical University.

Toyokawa, Satoshi, Chie Kanetou, Kazuo Inoue, and Yasuki Kobayashi [豊川智之他, 兼任千恵, 井上和男, 小林廉毅]. 2007. "医学部・医科大学設立後の医師供給の変化に関する検討 [Study on Changes in the Supply of Doctors, Medical University School of Medicine, after the Establishment]." 厚生の指標 [Health Index] 54 (13): 1–6.

7 Western Influences on Health Science Education in Korea: Medical, Nursing, and Public Health Education

OkRyun Moon

A Brief History of Western Influences on Korean Medical Education

Traditional Asian medicine dates back over two thousand years. But in the seventeenth century, Korean scholars began to analyze, experiment with, synthesize, and apply new medical knowledge arising from Ming China and from both Asian and Western medical practices. In the Joseon Dynasty, scholar Yi-Ik (1681–1763) analyzed the writings of the German Jesuit missionary Adam Schall von Bell on human anatomy and physiology in his famous *Seongho Saseol* (Mr. Seongho's Discourses on the Minute) and introduced Korea to contemporary Western medicine. Similar introductions of Western medicine followed— and even debates over its efficacy, in the case of Yi's *Seoguk-ui* (The Medicine of Western Countries)—in the writings of eighteenth-century scholars like Yi Gyu-gyeong and Pak Ji-won. Polymath Jeong Yak-yong (1762–1836) later used Western medicine as a lens to critique traditional Korean medicine (Yeo et al. 2012). But while Yi-Ik and other pioneers focused on the facts and theory of contemporary Western medicine, they did not address actual clinical practices. A more detailed investigation of these practices would take place in the nineteenth century, as Korea and East Asia came to renegotiate their relations with the West.

Western Medicine as a Byproduct of Foreign Trade

In 1637, the Joseon Dynasty lost its war with the Manchus (who would, within the following seven years, defeat Ming China, and establish the Qing Dynasty), and Korea was compelled to maintain a closed-door policy toward most trade outside of East Asia. In response to Western encroachments elsewhere in Asia, Daewongun (regent from 1863 to 1873) acted to strengthen this isolationist policy. Nonetheless, many Japanese traders began to take up residence in designated areas of port cities like Busan, due to the region's historical role in overseas trade and its geographical proximity to Japan.

In 1872, the Japanese doctor Takada Eisaku (高田英策) opened a private clinic in Choryang-jin to treat Japanese traders residing there (Ki 1996). With the Japan-Korea Treaty of 1876, trade between the two countries expanded and there were sharp increases in the number of Japanese merchants traveling to Korea and of Japanese residents in Korea. With those changes, modern Western medicine came to be more frequently practiced in Korea, primarily for the purpose of caring for the Japanese there.

This was an era of imperial competition over East Asia, and Japan's military was increasingly visible in Korea, including in the medical sector. The Japanese Navy established the Jesaeng Clinic (濟生醫院) in Busan in 1876 and Saengsaeng Clinic (生生醫院) in Wonsan in 1880, while the Japanese Army opened Kyeongseong Clinic (京城醫院) in Hanseong (today's Seoul, then the capital of Joseon) in 1880 and Incheon-Ilbon Clinic (仁川日本醫院) in Inchon in 1883 (Ki 1996). Administration of Busan's Jesaeng Clinic was transferred to the Japanese Army in April 1883, and then to the Japanese Settlement Corporation in 1885, changing its name from Jesaeng Clinic to Gongsaeng Clinic (共生醫院), then to Japanese Public Hospital (日本公立病院), and finally to Military Hospital (兵站病院) in 1894. When the First Sino-Japanese War broke out over control of the Korean peninsula in 1894, it opened a period of international and domestic unrest, with repercussions that affected the practice of medicine in Korea.

Missionary Care of the Sick at Jejungwon—Korea's First Modern National Hospital

In September 1884, Dr. Horace N. Allen came to Korea as an American missionary physician dispatched by the Northern Presbyterian Church. He served as a doctor based out of US diplomatic quarters, and he also took care of other foreign diplomats in Korea as a commissioned physician. Only a few months after his arrival, during the December 1884 Gapsin Coup, Allen gained fame for saving the life of Min Yeong-Ik, the nephew of the Queen. Min was severely wounded in the violence of the coup—in which a group of pro-Japanese activists staged a violent takeover of the Joseon government before being suppressed by Chinese troops—and under Allen's care, Min made a full recovery within three months. Having gained the confidence of the royal family, Allen wrote a letter to King Gojong through American envoy G. C. Foulk, proposing the construction of a national hospital (Yeo 2012; Ki 1997):

> As a American citizen, I would be glad to do all I can for the Corean people, and if the Government would grant me a few facilities, I think they would be amply repaid by having their sick cared for according to Western Science, and by having a place for wounded soldiers to be attended to. Also it would be the means of instructing young men in Western Medical and Sanitary Science. I am willing to take charge of one under the Government and not charge for my

services. All that would be necessary would be to provide a large Corean house in a healthy locality, with an annual appropriation for running expenses.... Should this be granted, the institution should be called "His Corean Majesty's" and it would certainly be gratifying to His Majesty to see his people cared for properly in their distress, while it would undoubtedly still further endear the people to their monarch and elevate them in many ways. (Seoul National University Hospital History and Cultural Center 2009, 21)

The king accepted the proposal and the Jejungwon (濟衆院, also known as the Institute for Aiding the Masses) was established (Seoul National University Hospital History and Cultural Center 2009). This was the first national hospital practicing Western medicine in Korea, and Dr. Allen worked there as a salaried physician.

Twenty Korean patients visited Jejungwon for medical consultations when it opened on April 9, 1885, according to Allen's record, and within ten days, the number of patients increased to around fifty a day. In 1886, nearly ten thousand Koreans received outpatient consultations and surgeries. Most of the outpatients were suffering from acute infectious and parasitic diseases: malaria was the leading disease (1,061 cases), followed by dermatitis (845 cases), syphilis (760 cases), eye diseases (629 cases), indigestion (58 cases), and epilepsy (307 cases) (Seoul National University Hospital History and Cultural Center 2009).

From the outset, Jejungwon was conceived as a teaching hospital. By March 1886, Allen had secured government funding and promises of medical employment of students and established the Medical Training Center at Jejungwon. The center taught English, basic sciences, medical techniques, pharmacy, and patient care to a handful of students. After Allen's departure from the hospital, three foreign medical missionary doctors—John W. Heron, C. C. Vinton, and Oliver R. Avison—served successively at Jejungwon, providing medical care and teaching students from 1887 onward. However, the majority of its students did not go on to serve in the medical profession (Ki 1997; Seoul National University Hospital History and Cultural Center 2009; Yeo et al. 2012).

Desperately low in funds after the Sino-Japanese War of 1894–1895, the Korean government decided to transfer administrative rights over Jejungwon to Oliver Avison, the hospital's director at the time, who transformed the institution into a Presbyterian missionary hospital (Choi 1996). With funds donated by Louis H. Severance in 1904, Avison upgraded the hospital's facilities, relaunching it at Severance Hospital in 1906.

Jejungwon represented the beginning of an explosion in the influence of Western medicine in Korea. The US Protestant Mission established hospitals in Busan, Pyongyang, Daegu, Suncheon, and other areas in the period 1891–1901 (Yeo et al. 2012). In October 1887, Boguyeogwan (普救女館 [Caring for and Saving Women Hospital]) opened under Methodist auspices, while the Lillian

Harris Memorial Hospital for Children (Dongdaemun Hospital) was opened in Seoul's East Gate area by missionary Dr. Rosetta Sherwood, who had arrived in Korea in 1890. (Dongdaemun Hospital later became the Ewha Womans Hospital College of Medicine, as it is known today.) In Pyongyang, Sherwood's husband, Dr. William James Hall, devoted himself to medical missionary work from 1891.

Western Medical Schools in the Joseon Dynasty

After Jejungwon's transfer to Presbyterian administration, the institution worked in conjunction with the government of the newly formed Great Korean Empire (1897–1910) to establish the Uihakgyo (Medical School) in 1899. This was the first free, official school for the study of Western medicine in Korea. A Western-style undergraduate medical curriculum was used to instruct the inaugural class of fifty-three students in sixteen subjects: zoology, botany, physics, chemistry, anatomy, physiology, drugs, diagnosis, internal medicine, surgery, ophthalmology, maternal and child health, hygiene, forensic medicine, immunization, and physical exercise. The medical school graduated its first class of nineteen certified doctors in 1902.

In 1902, the school opened an affiliated hospital called Gwangjewon (廣濟院, House of Extending Helpfulness). Smallpox vaccination and sanitation activities were major concerns at the time, and provision of medical care at the hospital was mostly shared with Japanese physicians who had been invited by the Joseon government (Seoul National University Hospital History and Cultural Center 2009). Nursing education also began at this time. Meanwhile, the Doctors' Association—the precursor of what would much later become the Korean Medical Association—was formed under the leadership of the Uihakgyo's Kim Ik-nam (Korean Medical Association).

Joseon's Western Medical Education and Traditional Medicine Begin to Develop in Tandem

Korean medicine had long developed under the influence of traditional Chinese medicine (Yeo et al. 2012). But as its center of gravity began to shift from traditional Korean herbal medicine to Western medicine, the former had to adapt accordingly. In response to the establishment of the Medical School (Uihakgyo), traditional herbal doctors demanded the establishment of their own medical school. Thus, the Joseon government chartered the Dongje School (同濟學校) in 1906, supported by the royal family, to teach both traditional herbal medicine and Western medicine (Lee and Ki 1996). In the pharmaceutical sector, drugs for topical application, powdered medications for coughs, and tonics for aiding digestion were produced by combining the philosophy of traditional Asian medicine with Western technologies and these drug formulas were widely used as emergency home remedies in Korea, while some traditional herbal doctors built Western-style clinics and pharmacies.

Daehan Hospital under the Early Japanese Regime

The Eulsa Treaty of 1905 established a Japanese protectorate over Korea, and the experience of Uihakgyo Gwangjewon (formerly known as Jejungwon) during this period is illustrative of Japanese interventions into Korean medicine. After the revision of its governing regulations in late December 1907, the institution came fully under the control of Japanese administrators and the Japanese military doctor Sato Susumu (佐藤進) was appointed as its director. In 1908, Uihakgyo Gwangjewon and the Red Cross Hospital (Jeoksipja Byeongwon) consolidated their disparate facilities into one comprehensive government hospital (Ki 1997). The new entity—a combined medical education, research, and treatment facility with authority over national medical provision efforts—was renamed Daehan Hospital, and on October 24, 1908, the opening ceremony of Daehan Medical School was held. Upon Korea's annexation by Japan in 1910, Daehan Hospital became the Government-General's Hospital. Minister of Internal Affairs Lee Chi-yong served concurrently as the first director of the hospital, and the staff comprised both Korean and Japanese doctors (Korea Health and Development Institute 2013). As Japanese control over the Korean peninsula increased in these years, so too did Japanese control over Daehan Hospital.

Hospital Resources under Japanese Colonial Rule

From its formal annexation of Korea in 1910 until the end of World War II in 1945, the Japanese colonial government managed medicine and medical education in Korea. The colonial administration, concerned with maintaining a healthy labor population, standardizing and increasing medical service provision, controlling epidemics such as smallpox, and demonstrating the efficacy of its rule, acted to curtail traditional Korean medicine while establishing Western-style hospitals and clinics as part of a public health regime (Han 1997). These developments reflected earlier changes in Meiji Japan—described in chapter 6 of this volume—in which the government acted to displace traditional Asian medicine with Western medicine in the German tradition (Lee and Ki 1996).

Despite these changes, however, an acute shortage of health facilities in Korea persisted throughout the colonial period and medical care remained inadequate and divided along lines of class and nationality. As shown in Table 7.1, after two decades of colonial rule, Korea had just 123 hospitals, equivalent to 6 percent of the total number of hospitals in Japan. Moreover, Korean hospitals served nearly six times the number of patients per hospital and areas ten times the size of their counterparts in Japan. This spurred the growth of a profit-driven private medical sector, with some 105 privately owned hospitals by 1940 (Han 1997).

Table 7.1. Comparisons of Hospital Resources in Colonial Korea and Japan in 1930.

	Korea (A)	Japan (B)	A/B	(B/A)
Population	21,058,305	64,450, 005	0.33	(3.1)
Number of Hospitals	123	2,128	0.06	
Population/Hospital	171, 213	30,286	5.7	(1/6)
Total Area	220,850	382,309.0	0.58	
	(in million m^2)	(in million m^2)		
Area/Hospital	1,794.6	179.6	10.0	(1/10)
	(in million m^2)	(in million m^2)		

Source: Data from Seoul National University Hospital History and Culture Center 2009.

In terms of medical education, the colonial government rolled back the teaching arm of Daehan Hospital, cutting student support, downgrading the institution, reevaluating curriculum, and changing the teaching language, among other measures (Park 2004). It then acted to standardize and control professional education in all fields through ordinances and charters. After six years of such changes, the training facility of the Government-General's Hospital was reestablished as Gyeongsung Professional Medical School (京城醫學專門學校) in 1916. Ten years later, in 1926, Gyeongsung Imperial University Medical College (京城帝國大學醫學部) was created. After Korea regained independence in 1945, these two schools would merge to become Seoul National University Medical College (SNUMC) and play an instrumental role in reshaping Korean medical education in the postwar period, but their role during the colonial era focused primarily on increasing the number of general practitioners in the country, not on training the next generation of medical researchers or professors.

Brief Overview of the Growth of Medical Schools in Post-Independence Korea

Under Japanese colonial rule, five universities—three private (Yonsei, Korea, and Ewha) and two public (Kyung-Puk and Chonnam)—had begun to operate their own medical colleges in the southern areas of Korea. (Yonsei had its roots in the Medical Training Center at Jejungwon, whose establishment in 1886 is discussed earlier in this chapter.) Despite the mounting medical care needs that accompanied the postindependence period, only three new medical colleges were built in Korea over a fourteen-year period, due mainly to social unpreparedness and financial difficulties. These included two public colleges, Seoul National University (created from Gyeongsong Professional Medical College and Gyeongsong Imperial Medical College) and Pusan National University, and one private college, Catholic University. Korea's medical infrastructure suffered further during the devastation of the Korean War (1950–1953), and while all of South Korea's medical schools continued to educate students, they were forced to operate under limited circumstances. The situation began to change in autumn 1952, as UN medical staff began to take part in training students and Korean medical schools, notably Daegu Medical College, began to regain and restore their physical plants (Steger 1953). International medical educational exchange, along with investments in medical infrastructure, marked the rest of the decade.

South Korea's remarkable economic expansion began in the 1960s, and that growth enabled the country to build eleven more medical colleges over the course of fifteen years (1961–1976). Korea's Fourth Five-Year Economic Development Plan, launched in 1977, gave greater weight to social development, including the medical needs of the burgeoning population. Twelve new medical colleges were established between 1977 and 1989, and the Korean National Health Insurance Program, introduced in 1989, marked a watershed in health care. Since 1990, the medical needs of the aging population and the demand for higher education have risen and an additional ten medical schools have been established, for a total of forty-one medical colleges (ten national and thirty-one private), or one medical school per 1.2 million people. (Table 7.2, below, illustrates the increase in medical colleges in Korea by historical period as described above.)

However, since the establishment of Gachon College of Medical Science in 1998, no new medical schools have been established. The Korean Medical Association (KMA)—the representative body of Korea's physicians—strongly opposes an increase in the number of medical colleges for fear of diluting the incomes of medical practitioners and the quality of medical education. It argues that Korea's current ratio of practitioners to population compares favorably with those of other Organization for Economic Cooperation and Development (OECD) countries (Korean Medical Association). Moreover, changes in the medical school accreditation system, the higher education system in general, and medical education pedagogy have created an environment in which further establishment of medical schools is contingent on broader consensuses in the medical field, in government, and in society.

Expansion of American Medical Education in South Korea

Starting with the 1945 liberation from Japan and beginning of US military occupation, South Korea's medical education system began to draw on American medical education approaches and methodology. American medicine and medical education were not new in Korea, but the roles that they played were significantly altered in the colonial period, and US and missionary influence in Korea were drastically curtailed during the Pacific War. This changed after 1945: American medical textbooks were introduced in 1947, clinical clerkships in 1957, internship programs in 1958, residency programs in 1959, and integrated courses in 1971. The

Table 7.2. Number of Medical Colleges in South Korea, from 1910 to 2014.

Years	Period	Number of New Medical Colleges Number (% of total)	Representative Schools
1910–1945 (35 years)	Colonial period	5 (12.2)	Yonsei, Kyung-Puk Korea, Chonnam, Ewha
1946–1960 (14 years)	Post-independence	3 (7.3)	SNU, Catholic, Pusan.
1961-1976 (15 years)	Economic development plans	11 (26.8)	Kyunghee, Chosun, Chung-nam, Hanyang, Chun-Puk, Jung-Ang, etc.
1977–1989 (13 years)	Social development	12 (29.3)	Wonju, Youngnam Sunchunhyang, Inje, Gyemyung, Kosin, etc.
1990–2014 (25 years)	After universal health coverage	10 (24.4)	Aju, Daegu-Catholic, Konyang, Kwandong, etc.
Total		41 (100)	

Source: Date compiled by author.

lecture-based Japanese-style of medical education shifted toward the contemporary American model, which emphasized clinical practice and experimentation. At the same time, a number of cooperative projects, personnel exchanges, and technological transfers—such as the Minnesota Project at Seoul National University (also known as the SNU Cooperative Project) and the Memorial Chest Surgery Hospital and General Ward Hospital at Yonsei University Medical Center—worked to restore the physical and intellectual infrastructure of Korean medical education in the postwar era (Kim and Hwang 2000; Yonsei University Health System 2009).

In 1975, with the need for teacher training programs for health care workers on the rise, the National Teachers Training Center (NTTC) was established at Seoul National University Medical College with the assistance of the World Health Organization (WHO) and China Medical Board (CMB). NTTC aimed at improving the quality of continuing education for health care nationwide, and at SNUMC, it bolstered the professional development of health science faculty at the School of Medicine, Dentistry, Nursing and Public Health through workshops, seminars, and other educational programming. It is estimated that over a thirty-seven-year period, from 1975 to 2012, NTTC hosted over 450 workshops and trained over fifteen thousand medical professionals (Kang, 2013).

The administrators of Korea's various medical institutions formed organizations to set the direction for medical education, make policy recommendations to the government, and share information. An Association of Deans of Medical Colleges had existed since the 1960s, and following growth in its membership and scope of activities, it became the Korean Association of Medical Education in 1971 (later the Korean League of Medical Education [KLME]). In 1984, KLME members established the Korean League of Deans of Medical Colleges in an effort to refocus membership on medical school administrators and to address the issues pertinent to administration, curriculum, funding, and educational policy (Korean Association of Medical Education 2010). These organizations, in turn, focused throughout the 1980s and 1990s on pedagogical development and reform in medical education. Seeking to facilitate active, student-centered learning, medical schools began to introduce problem-based learning (PBL) and the Objective Structured Clinical Examination (OSCE) into their curriculums in the 1990s (Kim and Kee 2012). This has resulted in higher levels of medical student success and satisfaction.

The number of medical schools in South Korea more than tripled from the 1970s to the 1990s (see Appendix 1), making quality control a more pressing issue. Gaps in medical education standards and quality had arisen between older medical schools (e.g., Yonsei and SNUMC) and newly established ones (e.g., Seonam Medical School and Kwandong), as evidenced by the number of faculty, by the curriculums, and by the quality of the affiliated teaching hospitals.

The Accreditation Board of Medical Education (ABME) was established in 1997 to address these issues. It was intended to provide a means for the medical profession itself to evaluate and improve basic and clinical medical education. The independence of ABME is significant: it was established in response to a 1996 attempt by the Ministry of Education to evaluate and rank medical schools that was widely deemed unproductive in the medical education community. ABME later expanded its scope to cover the lifelong professional education of medical doctors, becoming the Korean Institute of Medical Education and Evaluation (KIMEE) in 2003. Aimed at universal participation and quality improvement in Korean medical education, ABME's first accreditation round of 2000–2005 drew on global standards that had been tailored to and piloted in the most recently established institutions in Korea. Since 2007, KIMEE has used the accreditation process to promote benchmarking and raise quality in key areas in an attempt to bring Korean medical education more in line with the best practices across the world (Ahn and Ahn 2014).

The Korean medical education field is now working on multiple fronts to improve students' research and patient care abilities. The roles of patients are becoming more central in the contemporary provision of medical care, and Korean medical schools have joined their peers around the world in implementing patient-doctor-society courses (PDS), clinical performance examinations (CPX), and medical simulation centers within their curriculums since the 2000s

(Makoul and Schofield 1999; Haidet et al. 2006). Additionally, in the fall of 2009, the Korean Society of Medical Education and the National Health Personnel Licensing Examination Board responded to the ongoing debates in Korea and the United States on how best to assess the "skills and attitude" of clinicians by adding a clinical skills test (CST), along with a written examination, to the medical licensing examination (Lee 2008). Preliminary surveys indicate that this has created more confident, communicative, and competent medical students and interns, though some scholars have noted that the rubric for passing remains to be calibrated and that the long-term effects of these additions on reducing errors or increasing patient satisfaction have yet to be measured (Park 2012). Medical education has been further enriched through the linkage of professors' mentoring services and student research activities (Yena and Lee 2013). Writing a thesis is now a graduation requirement for the fulfillment of the bachelor's degree at medical colleges.

Two Major External Influences on the Development of Contemporary Medicine in the Republic of Korea

American medicine has played a predominant role in the structuring of medical education in postwar Korea. The examples below highlight the work of two entities that were fundamental in initiating and shaping the processes of postwar exchange between US and Korean medical practitioners and institutions in the twentieth century—the Minnesota Project (1954–1961) and the China Medical Board (1953–1989).

The Minnesota Project

The Minnesota Project, officially titled the Seoul National University Cooperative Project, was a large-scale education assistance program run by the US International Cooperation Administration (ICA) under the US Department of State between 1954 and 1961. The project's purpose was to stimulate the development of medical faculty members, the improvement of medical research and education, the renovation of facilities, and technological transfer between the United States and Korea. The project began with collaboration between the University of Minnesota and the SNU Colleges of Medicine, Engineering, and Agriculture and was later extended to include the School of Public Administration (DiMoia 2013).

Much has been written regarding the impact of the Minnesota Project on Korean medicine in the form of semiannual progress reports, and even of a doctoral dissertation (Lee 2006). According to these reports, seventy-seven SNU medical faculty members studied at the University of Minnesota either on three-month observation tours or by attending three- or four-year degree programs. Fifty-nine foreign advisors—including eleven medical school advisors—were stationed at SNU for consultations on matters ranging from clinical care to hospital administration. The total project cost approximately US $10 million, including the cost of faculty exchanges and construction of facilities and the purchase of educational materials.

The Minnesota Project introduced radical changes within South Korean medical education, such as the clinical clerkship and intern and residency training programs. Cutting-edge clinical techniques, such as open heart surgery, were introduced and modified in Korean medical education nearly concurrently with their development in Minnesota. A generation of Korean physicians established international networks of technical and material exchange, and the educational standards and pedagogical methods of medicine and nursing in Korea were transformed (Kim and Hwang 2000). The decision to run the project in cooperation with Seoul National University—as opposed to with a wider range of partners—had been made in order to concentrate resources for maximum effect and under the assumption that the national university, in its capacity as a leading institution and as a government affiliate, would be best able to disseminate the program's benefits through future personnel appointments and standard-setting. Despite challenges and unintended consequences, such as brain drain, the Minnesota Project has been credited for bringing a "drastic and rapid change" to the Seoul National University medical curriculum, which, in turn, became the archetype of medical education and research in the Republic of Korea (Stoddard 1959; Kim and Hwang 2000).

China Medical Board Grants

The China Medical Board left China in 1951, and by 1953, it had determined that, until it was feasible to return, its best course of action was to fund medical education programs in other Asian countries. CMB made its first grant to a Korean institution, Kyung-Puk University, in 1953, and it continued to invest heavily in South Korea throughout the postwar period. In fact, from 1953 to 1989, it awarded more than US $11.8 million in grants in to South Korean institutions (7.8 percent of total CMB grant funds for the 1951–2000 period). Seven Korean institutions were recipients of CMB grants: Chonnam University Medical College, Ewha Medical College, Kyung-Puk University, Pusan National University, Seoul National University, Sudo Medical College, and Yonsei University Medical College (Norris 2003).

South Korea's needs and CMB's priorities in this period can be seen in the allocation of grants: the top categories were faculty development, at 22 percent, capital projects (for construction and physical plant development), at 20 percent, and biomedical research, at 14 percent (see Figure 7.1). The second tier of CMB grants in South Korea comprised investments in basic teaching infrastructure for educating medical professionals, sustainable general endowment funds, and library materials. From 1951, when CMB left China, to 2000, South Korea accounted for large swaths of total CMB grants in the areas of capital projects (30 percent), nursing education (15 percent), library development (10 percent), and faculty development (9 percent) (Norris 2003).

Two institutions were the recipients of most of this funding: Seoul National University received just over $6.1 million, accounting for 54 percent of CMB's Korean grants, and Yonsei Medical College, with nearly $4.6 million, accounted for 41 percent. Data compiled from the annual financial reports of CMB also reveal that—as opposed to their fellow South Korean grantee institutions, which received more time- or category-specific investments—these two institutions were the targets of a variety of grants, reflecting both the changing needs of South Korea in a period of economic and demographic transition and the evolving priorities in CMB grant-making in the latter half of the twentieth century (for more on this, see chapter 1 in this volume).

Yonsei Medical College received the lion's share of capital projects funding—18 percent, in fact, of total CMB grants made in this category throughout East Asia in the latter half of the twentieth century—whereas SNUMC received around six times the amount of grants that Yonsei did for medical curriculum development and over twice the amount of Yonsei's for faculty development. Through its support of SNUMC, CMB played a key role in the development of Korean medical education.

Initial funding for SNUMC was provided for the purchase of medical journals—sixty-four journals with ten-year subscriptions, worth $1,500 annually. In 1963, after the completion of the Minnesota Project, Dr. Sejin Rha, dean of SNUMC at the time, requested CMB assistance in finding a medical education consultant who could help solve the college's administrative and educational problems. CMB subsequently recruited Dr. N. J. Gault, who had previously served as an advisor to the Minnesota Project at SNUMC, and it increased its assistance to the medical school, continuing to fund the purchasing of books and journals for the medical library while expanding its scope to medical school equipment and supplies, visiting professorships, fellowships for SNUMC faculty to study in the United States (forty-four in total), and research grants. In this sense, when the Minnesota Project came to a close in 1961, CMB effectively took over its objectives, continuing to develop faculty members and improve medical research and education (China Medical Board 1951–1989).

Arguably the most influential contribution of Minnesota Project and CMB grants in South Korea was the establishment of a system of high quality education for health professionals—including physicians, nurses, and public health practitioners—through faculty development fellowships, assistance for infrastructure and facilities development, and support to health sciences research. While the Minnesota Project's development assistance kick-started these efforts, grant support from CMB helped to fortify and sustain medical, nursing, and public health education in Korea.

170 | *Medical Education in East Asia*

CMB Grants to South Korea 1951-1989 (Percentage by Category)

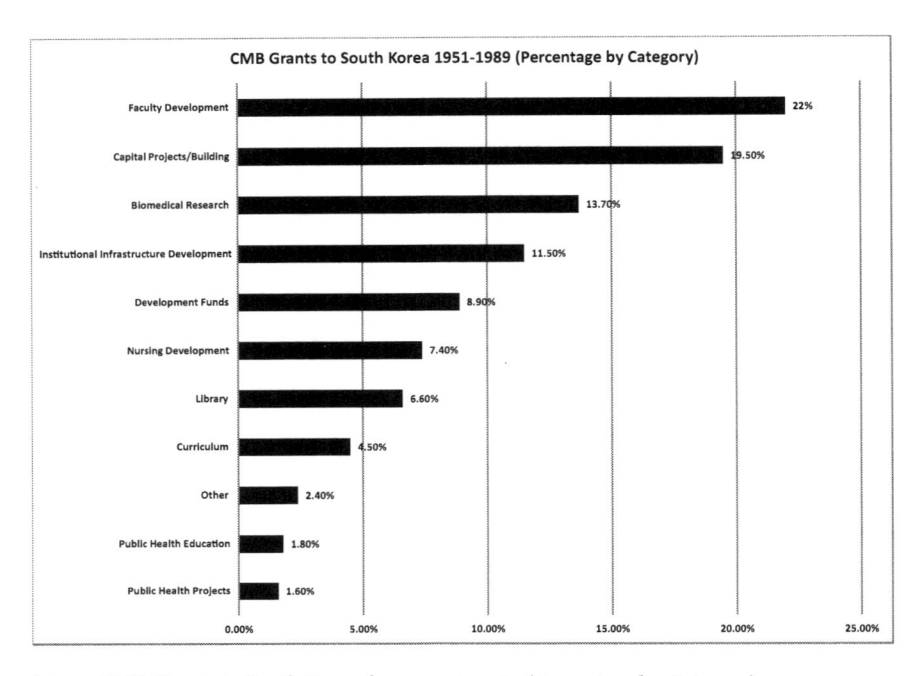

Category	Percentage
Faculty Development	22%
Capital Projects/Building	19.50%
Biomedical Research	13.70%
Institutional Infrastructure Development	11.50%
Development Funds	8.90%
Nursing Development	7.40%
Library	6.60%
Curriculum	4.50%
Other	2.40%
Public Health Education	1.80%
Public Health Projects	1.60%

Fig. 7.1 CMB Grants to South Korea from 1951 to 1989 (Percentage by Category). *Source*: Data from China Medical Board 1950–2006.

While both projects focused on improving the quality of medical education in South Korea, perhaps the most significant difference between the two may be found in the way in which matching funds were administered. From the outset, CMB required individual universities—the beneficiaries of its grants—to allocate matching funds in order to receive assistance. In contrast, the Korean government itself was responsible for matching funds to SNUMC during the Minnesota Project. At the time, Korea was not accustomed to a culture of contribution, but CMB's requirement of matching grants spurred medical schools to create these important funds, which became research foundations for public health and medical science education. In this respect, CMB matching funds prompted medical schools in South Korea to take the initiative in generating educational and research funds. This remains central to the future capabilities of South Korean health care and health sciences.

Current Status of Medical Education in South Korea

This section examines the current landscape of South Korea's medical education system and identifies trends that will serve as the basis for considering the prospects for Korean medical education in the concluding section of this chapter.

From an ODA Recipient to Donor

South Korea has succeeded in transitioning from an official development assistance (ODA) recipient country to an ODA donor country, and it joined the OECD's Development Assistance Committee (DAC) in December 2009. Its medical education field now implements best practices at a similar pace as its peers throughout the world. Korea is also in a position to move beyond simply adopting standards and technologies in medical education to modifying and creating them. In this task, Korea is poised to draw on its own rich history of forging a medical education system out of differing influences and under disparate and often difficult circumstances—lessons of value to other countries throughout the world.

National Teacher Training in a Post-Developmental Korea

The National Teachers Training Center (NTTC) strengthened medical education according to the recommendations of the WHO, hosting hundreds of workshops and seminars to build networks for the dissemination of standardized knowledge about teaching, evaluation, and curriculum to thousands of health education faculty. The center has also functioned as a regional education development center (REDC) before and since its incorporation into the J. W. Lee Center for Global Medicine (established in 2010), and it remains active in linking and training the faculty leadership of medical colleges throughout Korea.

However, the role, mission, and reach of the NTTC/J. W. Lee Center—and of national teacher training in general—have been changing since the 1990s. This comes in response to the high level of development South Korea has achieved since the late 1980s, the slowdown in the establishment of new medical colleges since the 1990s, the increasing complexity and sophistication of the medical field's governing and accreditation arrangements, and the country's transition from global aid recipient to global aid donor. Specialized organizations within the medical education field, such as the Accreditation Board of Medical Education created in 1996 (later changed to the Korean Institute of Medical Education and Evaluation in 2003), have taken over some of the functions previously within the NTTC's purview. The mission statement and activities of the J. W. Lee Center indicate a shift in perspective, from inside Korea to outside Korea. The "Projects" portion of the center's webpage shows forty-one projects underway in Southeast Asia and Mongolia, versus thirty underway within Korea (J. W. Lee Center).

Rocky Shifts in Curriculum Structure

Korean medical education has been experimenting with changes in its curriculum structure with largely mixed results, in terms of student and school satisfaction, student specialization choice, and availability of medical care. Most of

Korea's forty-one medical schools have joined their peers around the world in integrating student-centered pedagogy, such as problem-based learning (PBL) and block lectures, and in using objective-structured clinical examinations (OSCE) and clinical performance examinations (CPX) to teach and improve clinical skills. Korean medical schools are also developing and sharing online learning resources through a consortium of e-learning in medical education. While these developments have not been without their challenges, recent research suggests that the trouble spots are quite easily pinpointed and that the overall effect of their adoption so far has been positive (Kim et al. 2009).[1]

Until recently, however, the structure of Korea's medical education curriculum has been quite static. The system consisted of a six-year curriculum structure in which undergraduate students took general elective and basic science courses in the first two years and preclinical courses for the next two years and, finally, did two years of clinical clerkships. This structure is now undergoing a degree of change. Most notably, medical schools have been experimenting with a shift from the standard entry program (SEP)—through which medical students were selected upon high school graduation and entered medical school as first-year undergraduates—to a graduate entry program (GEP) similar to that in the United States.

However, this experiment appears to have been a failure. The majority of medical schools that changed to GEP programs have since switched back to the six-year SEP. The reasons include the GEP system's exacerbation of the existing trend toward specialization among students, the additional hardships its length imposes on prospective students, and confusion over just what improvements GEP offers over SEP.[2] Furthermore, after finishing medicine graduate programs, new doctors have continued to cluster their practices in the Seoul-Gyeonggi Province area, worsening the existing poor distribution of human resources. Students were unhappy that the graduate programs cost much more than the undergraduate programs and that the length of study had been expanded from six years to eight years (Hwang and Choi 2010). As of December 2013, only five medical schools (Konkuk, Dongguk, Kangwon, Cheju, and CHA Medical) have continued to offer graduate programs.

Most graduate medical school alumni must go through a one-year internship and three or four more years of resident training for their career development, depending on their specialty. Although all graduates are qualified for general practice, this process of specialization has resulted in an acute shortage of general practitioners, who make up only about 10 percent of the total pool of physicians. Additionally, the requirement that Korean men complete twenty-one to thirty-six months of mandatory military service has been one of the main obstacles to introducing graduate medical programs, as it discourages male students from wanting to enter into lengthy graduate programs. This situation is further complicated by the fact that public health care in regional areas relies heavily on the male medical college students assigned to these hospitals as part of their military service. Thus, with fewer males entering medical school or beginning their medical training as college graduates—having already completed military service in nonmedical capacities—the shortage in human resources in provincial public health care is becoming all the more acute (Kim 2014). In the final analysis, few seem to be satisfied with the change to the eight-year graduate medical programs in South Korea.

Emphasis on Continuing Medical Education and Evaluation

Korea's Medical Service Act (Article 30, Paragraphs 2–3) stipulates that the "medical personnel shall attend refresher training" conducted by a "central association." (Medical Service Act, 2011, Article 30, Paragraphs 2–3), and the Korean Medical Association requires its members to complete ten hours of continuing education annually (Korea Medical Association). CME has been included in Korean law since the mid-twentieth century, but it only emerged as an issue in the early 1980s, with the Korean government and the KMA instituting structured methods for carrying out this legal provision. In the early 1990s, the KMA responded to the increasing amount and availability of breakthrough medical research—as well as to the globalizing medical education and treatment markets—by establishing an annual roundtable on the matter of CME (Kim 2004). CME has grown into a widely practiced and diverse component of Korean medical education, but its success in increasing the quality of medical care has been tempered by recent problems with participation levels, as well as by criticism of the effectiveness and relevance of its content, the degree of quality control, and the level of fiscal and academic support for CME as a whole (Kim 2004; Yoo 2006).

A range of options is available to physicians for obtaining CME credits, including lectures, workshops, conferences, journal publications, online courses, and so on. At present, most medical schools are equipped with medical education units that provide support for teaching activities, curriculum design, faculty development, and conducting medical education research. Yet, improving the coordination between the KMA, these education units, and the hospitals employing doctors around the improvement and implementation of CME remains a priority in Korean medical education.

Postgraduate education now forms a part of the KIMEE's regular accreditation assessment, which examines medical programs across the following six domains: (1) administrative systems, (2) educational objectives, (3) student support requirements, (4) faculty requirements, (5) educational facilities, and (6) postgraduate education. This assessment is done every five years, and specific evaluation criteria are reestablished in each evaluation period. Internally, the adoption of innovative teaching and learning methods in CME, as in basic medical education itself, continues to be a central concern of medical school administrations and faculties: PBL is on the rise, as is a student-centered pedagogy

(Jeong 2005). Student-centered learning becomes increasingly important in the CME environment, in which participants are already practitioners themselves. A shift to a competency-based educational approach, starting in the 1990s in Korea, has also enhanced the quality of medical education and emphasized patient-centered care. As a part of this shift, the top priorities for medical education—both continuing and basic—in Korea currently comprise medical ethics, communication skills of medical professionals, and professional competence (Kim 2004).

Exporting the Korean Health Sciences Education Model

Korea's recent transformation from ODA recipient nation to donor nation makes it well-suited to leadership in the development of global health care. In this role, Korea is able to draw on its own history of applying and modifying best practices in medical education under diverse circumstances and, more importantly, to build on some of the competitive advantages it has developed in health care and health education. In cooperation with global and national aid programs, developing countries in Africa and Southeast Asia—including Laos, Uganda, and Zimbabwe—are now importing portions of the Korean health services education model as well as Korean health care technologies, bringing Korea's experience of knowledge and technology transfer full circle. In the Dr. Lee Jong-Wook/Seoul National University Global Project, for example, we find a present-day version of the Minnesota Project, with SNUMC running exchange fellowships, surgical training programs, global health symposiums, and medical writing workshops. In 2011, SNUMC and the University of Health Sciences of Lao began a medical exchange program through which SNUMC provides medical equipment and training to Lao students. SNU's Lee Jong-Wook Seoul Global Center holds the International Symposium on Global Health each year to discuss ways to improve the health of peoples in Asia and Africa and, in the process, create and expand the kinds of personal and professional networks that made the Minnesota Project so groundbreaking (J. W. Lee Center).

These efforts suggest that Korea's experience with the Minnesota and CMB projects can serve as important models, not only for technological transfer, development, and exchange, but also in working through some of the challenges associated with these processes, including the laws and export frameworks of donor nations, the personal situations of the doctors participating in the exchanges, the economic and practical limitations to full technical transfer, and the relevance of diseases targeted and skills taught.[3]

Future Prospects

Four themes emerge in considering the future of Korean medical education: international leadership, domestic challenges, the outlook for international development, and the unique nexus of international and domestic factors on the divided Korean peninsula.

The Potential of Korea: Assuming a Leadership Role in the International Community

In many respects, South Korea's economic gains have extended into other sectors. Overall life expectancy is eighty-one years, an increase of some twenty-six years over the past four decades. The country has continued to advance its education, health, and insurance-based health care systems, achieving universal primary education and universal health care coverage ahead of many other developing countries.

South Korea has begun sharing its experiences and expertise with developing countries, and health sciences and education have played a key role in these efforts. Schools like the medical school of Kumi University in Uganda are now importing Korean medical education models (A. T. Ahn 2012). Meanwhile, Konkuk University has just signed a memorandum of understanding (MOU) with Zimbabwe Medical School in Harare regarding a transfer of technology for cardiac transplantation (E. Lee 2012). Hospital construction projects are taking place in Africa, Latin America, and Southeast Asia under Korean sponsorship.

Strategies for Dealing with Domestic Challenges

On the domestic front, Korea faces a range of challenges, including rapidly rising health care costs (nominally, a tenfold increase over the past twenty years,) a health care labor shortage (most notably, acute physician and nursing labor shortages), a rapid rise in the use of high-cost technologies (CT scans are 37.1 per every 1 million people and MRIs are 19 per every 1 million people), rising inpatient bed complements (in particular, the sustained rise in the number of chronic nursing care beds—the number of chronic nursing beds per every 1,000 persons was 17.24 for South Korea, while for Japan, France, and Sweden, these numbers were 12.16, 4.57, and 1.3, respectively), the ongoing experiment of transitioning the medical educational system from a six-year system to a "4+4" eight-year system like that in the United States, and the increasing social burden of dementia (currently 570,000 dementia patients, representing a two-fold increase over the past twenty years). These problems are closely related to the dominance of the private health care system, which makes up over 85 percent of both health care spending and of ownership of health resources (OECD/DAC Review Team 2008). Specific reform measures are needed, including strengthening public medical care in order to balance out the highly skewed privatized health care system and creating a national health promotion system focused on preventive health care.

Despite these problems, however, national health expenditures have been controlled at 6.9 percent of GDP, while maintaining high average life expectancy and low infant and maternal mortality rates, relative to other OECD countries (ibid.). The Conference Board of Canada evaluated the efficiency of the South Korean health system as fifth highest in the world. In evaluating this achievement, we should not overlook the role of the government in health promotion and prevention. In addition, Korea's schools of medicine, public health, and nursing have played an important advisory role, with many serving as consultants to the government in these efforts.

In order to overcome the domestic challenges to health care and medical education, however, both the role of the government and cooperation among academic institutions become more critical than ever before. Some of the major areas in which this cooperation is currently being called for or forged in revamping public health care include the following:

- solving the shortage of specialists at the thirty-four provincial/municipal hospitals by dispatching resident physicians as part of their specialty training at university hospitals;
- reforming the payment systems of providers, including Korean diagnosis-related groups (DRGs);
- changing the mass purchasing of drugs under national health insurance via the state marketplace;
- restructuring the long-term health care insurance system through fostering home health care;
- and correcting the lack of educational services for families struggling with dementia.

Beyond these specific policy debates, it is clear that medical, nursing, and public health education in general will need to be further adapted to meet the needs of a globalizing, urbanizing, and aging South Korean population in the years to come.

Cooperation with KOICA and KOFIH and Official Development Assistance

South Korea began offering aid in the form of credit assistance in 1987—the year of its democratization—with the creation of the Economic Developing Cooperation Fund (EDCF). This was followed by the establishment of the Korea International Cooperation Agency (KOICA) in 1991 (OECD/DAC Review Team 2008). South Korea's ODA in 2012 was equivalent to only 0.14 percent of its GNI, just half of the 2012 OECD average (0.29 percent). Even compared with ODA of countries of similar economic trading magnitude—for example the Netherlands and Australia—South Korea ranks lower, with the Netherlands contributing 0.71 percent of its GNI in 2012 and Australia 0.36 percent in the same year. However, South Korea's rate of increase in ODA has been quite steep compared to other countries. And, while both KOICA and the Korea Foundation for International Health (KOFIH) are relatively small organizations in terms of ODA amounts, they are known among recipient countries and among international donor agencies for having relatively fast decision-making processes.

Potential Medical Cooperation with North Korea

The division between South Korea and North Korea has lasted for over seventy years. North Korea is one of the poorest countries in the world, and its public health ranks among the worst in the world. It is isolated from the international community, and its government is unpredictable and dangerous. Yet, there have been efforts to initiate North-South cooperation in the health sector. A number of hospitals were built and supported in Pyongyang, North Korea's capital city, with assistance from South Korean individuals and nongovernmental organizations from the 1990s on, and transfers of medicines and medical technologies, and even visits by medical personnel, have occurred in the intervening years. It is hard to assess the relative impact of these efforts within the North Korean medical system as a whole. Meanwhile, legal restrictions and the deteriorating relations between the two from the mid-2000s onward continue to limit meaningful medical cooperation on the peninsula (Kim, Lee, and Lee 2013).

The need for this type of cooperation, however, remains great, and as a humanitarian cause, a renewed effort to expand and sustain this exchange is worthwhile. Initially, this might involve establishing emergency clinics, infirmaries, or dispensaries in the demilitarized zone (DMZ) and in joint economic zones, such as the Kaesong Industrial Complex, for free care for residents of North Korea. The recent reopening of dialogue between North and South on allowing reunions between elderly members of families separated by the national division provides a good opportunity to open such clinics. Were this kind of cooperation to occur, then future technological transfers, such as sending medical textbooks and medical equipment and supplies to North Korea, might be possible.

Conclusion

This chapter has traced the historical path of the development of medical education in Korea over the past several centuries, examining the different traditions of medical education—traditional Asian medicine, late-nineteenth-century Western missionary medicine, turn-of-the-twentieth-century German academic medicine, Japanese colonial public health, and mid-twentieth-century American biomedicine—that laid down roots on the peninsula. It reassessed two projects that remade the landscape of Korean medicine in the postwar era—the Minnesota Project (1954–1961) and the China Medical Board grants (1953–1989)—and opened new possibilities for international exchanges in medical education. It highlighted Korea's emerging role in international health care development as it directs portions of its overseas development assistance to medical education.

Yet, the kind of leadership role Korea will play in Northeast Asia remains to be seen. Certainly, the region is not without its cross-border cooperative efforts—particularly in terms of tracking and containing infectious diseases such as HIV/AIDS, dealing with migrant health, and creating societies of specialists (Japan Center for International Exchange 2006; Bom, Chung, and Lee 2011). The medical schools of the region could prove to be another avenue for cross-border cooperation. Given the fraught history of the region, this is, of course, not without its challenges. But in combining the differing experiences of each country and the comparative advantages each has gained in educating generations of medical professionals, greater possibilities emerge for improving public health and, perhaps, the stability of the region.

In a different era, the Indian poet Rabindranath Tagore elegantly wrote, "In the golden age of Asia / Korea was one of its lamp bearers / And that lamp is waiting to be lighted once again for the illumination of the East" (Tagore 2006, 97). As we have seen above, by leveraging its unique experiences with medical education development under diverse influences and in a range of contexts—from colonialism to war to nation-building—as well as its responsibilities as an ODA donor and negotiator of challenges that bridge the domestic-international divide, South Korea can, through effective international cooperation, indeed, be one of the bearers of light in Asia and the world in the century to come.

Appendix 7.1. List of Medical Colleges: Year of Establishment, Ownership, and Number of Total Graduates as of May 2002.

Year of Establishment	Name of University	Ownership: National (N) versus Private (P)	Total Graduates as of May 2002
1885	Yonsei	P	*
1933	Kyung-Puk	N	6,707
1938	Korea	P	6,045
1944	Chonnam	N	5,707
1945	Ewha Womans	P	3,165
1946	Seoul	N	8,212
1954	Catholic	P	3,713

Year of Establishment	Name of University	Ownership: National (N) versus Private (P)	Total Graduates as of May 2002
1955	Pusan	N	4,882
1965	Kyunghee	P	2,962
1966	Chosun	P	3,437
1968	ChoongNam	N	2,905
1968	Hanyang	P	3,040
1970	Chun-Puk	N	2,708
1971	Joong-Ang	P	2,290
1977	Yonsei (Wonju Campus)	P	1,673
1978	Soonchunhyang	P	1,813
1979	Inje	P	1,734
1979	Youngnam	P	1,477
1979	Gyemyung	P	1,393
1981	Wonkwang	P	1,322
1981	Kosin	P	1,123
1981	KyungSang	N	1,170
1982	Hanlim	P	1,082
1985	Inha	P	542
1985	Dong-A	P	575
1986	Dongguk	P	455
1986	Konkuk	P	385
1987	ChoongBuk	N	535
1988	Ulsan	P	241
1988	Dangoog	P	258
1988	Aju	P	256
1991	Daegu-Catholic	P	72
1995	Konyang	P	67
1995	Seonam	P	48
1995	Kwandong	P	62
1997	KangWon	N	52
1997	SungKyunKwan	P	*
1997	Pochun Joongmoon	P	32
1997	Ulji	P	*
1998	Gachon	P	*
1998	Cheju	N	23

*Data not available.
Source: Data compiled by author.

Notes

1. A more recent consideration of the preliminary benefits and challenges of this approach may be found in Hye Won Jang and Kyong-Jee Kim, "Use of Online Clinical Videos for Clinical Skills Training for Medical Students: Benefits and Challenges," BMC Medical Education 14:56 (2014). Last accessed August 15, 2016. https://bmcmededuc.biomedcentral.com/articles/10.1186/1472-6920-14-56. Here, Jang and Kim cite the preliminary challenges in using these videos as including limited adoption by professors and curriculum developers despite wide student use, lack of optimization for the mobile environments in which these materials are most often accessed, lack of wide consideration or dissemination of best practices in video production, and lack of interactivity in the materials.

2. Numerous studies have tried to ascertain the differences in the characteristics, motivations, experiences, and perceptions of GEP entrants versus their SEP counterparts and to make recommendations for future improvements in the GEP experience. See, e.g., Roh Hye Rin, "Differentiation Strategy of Graduate Entry Programme," Hanyang Medical Reviews 32.1 (2012): 17–24; J. J. Han et al., "The Comparison of Backgrounds and Characteristics of Students in Medical College and Graduate Medical School: A Case Study of One Medical School," Korean Journal of Medical Education 20.1 (2008): 11–12; and the articles in Korean Journal of Medical Education 21.2 (2009) by Hye Rin Roh et al. ("Multiple Mini-Interview in Selecting Medical Students"), Byung Kuk Lee et al. ("The Relationship between Empathy and Medical Education System, Grades, and Personality in Medical College Students and Medical School Students"), Eun-Kyung Chung et al ("Comparison of Learning Styles between Medical Students and Professional Graduate Medical School Students"), and Bong Sik Hing et al. ("Comparison of Patient-centeredness Changes between Medical School Graduate [Students] and Medical Students after Psychiatric Clerkship").

3. On considerations of the applicability of diseases targeted and the uncritical acceptance of skills taught, see Kim and Hwang (2000) and Wang-jun Lee (2006). Additionally, Young Moon Chae's recent discussion of the export of Korean health information systems raises the interesting question of how export agendas and medical laws affect technology transfer, as well as how the different needs of the health care authorities of countries like Mongolia and the Philippines lead them, in turn, to different institutions within Korean health care. This serves to remind us that, while we discuss Korean health care and health education in the aggregate here, the present situation is already one of a considerable level differentiation in expertise and global networks. See also Young Moon Chae, "Going Abroad of Korean Health Information Systems," Healthcare Information Research 20.3 (July 2014): 161–62.

References

Ahn, Alexander Tehoon. 2012. "Korean Professor Becomes Ugandan University President." Korea Times, April 23. Last accessed May 15, 2015. https://www.koreatimes.co.kr/www/news/include/print.asp?newsIdx=109562.

Ahn, E. and D. Ahn, 2014. "Beyond Accreditation: Excellence in Medical Education." Medical Teacher 36 (1): 84–85.

Bom, Hee-sung, June-Key Chung, and Myung-Chul Lee. 2011. "A Decade of the Asian Regional Cooperative Council for Nuclear Medicine: A Path to Reduce Heterogeneity of Nuclear Medicine Practice in Asia." World Journal of Nuclear Medicine 10 (2): 113–14.

Chae, Young Moon. 2014. "Going Abroad of Korean Health Information Systems." Healthcare Information Research 20 (3): 161–62.

China Medical Board of New York. 1950–2006. Accounting Records. New York: China Medical Board.
———. 1951–1989. *Meetings of the Board of Trustees Minutes*. New York: China Medical Board.
Choi, Je-chang. 1996. *Han-mi uihaksa: Uisa ui kil 60 nyeon eul dorabomyeo* [Korean-US Medical History: A Look Back at 60 Years as a Physician]. Seoul: Yeongnim Kadineol.
DiMoia, John P. 2013. *Reconstructing Bodies: Biomedicine, Health, and Nation-Building in South Korea Since 1945*. Stanford, CA: Stanford University Press.
Haidet, Paul, P. Adam Kelly, Susan Bentley, Benjamin Blatt, Calvin L. Chou, Auguste H. Fortin, VI, Geoffrey Gordon, Catherine Gracey, Heather Harrell, David S. Hatem, Drew Helmer, Debora S. Paterniti, Dianne Wagner, and Thomas S. Inui. 2006. "Not the Same Everywhere: Patient-Centered Learning Environments at Nine Medical Schools." *Journal of General Internal Medicine* 21 (5): 405–09.
Han, Gil Soo. 1997 "The Rise of Western Medicine and Revival of Traditional Medicine in Korea: A Brief History." *Korean Studies* 21: 96–121.
Hur, Yera, Kim Sun, and Keumho Lee. 2013. "What Kind of Mentoring Do We Need? A Review of Mentoring Program Studies for Medical Students." *Journal of Korean Medical Education* 25 (1): 5–13.
Hwang, Gyu-in and Yena Choi. 2010. "Uihak jeonmun daehakweon sasilsang silpae: uidae wa biseut hande hakbi ↑hyogwa ↓ . . . 'eojeongjjeong 6 nyeon donggeo' maknaeryeo [Graduate schools of medicine in reality a failure: similar to medical colleges, but tuition ↑ results ↓ . . . '6 years' noncommittal coexistence' comes to a close]." *Donga ilbo*, Education Section, July 2.
Iwamoto, Yasushi, Tadashi Fukui, Masako Ii, Hiroyuki Kawaguchi, Miki Kohara, and Makoto Saito. 2004. "Chapter 1: Healthcare Delivery and Financing in Japan, Korea and Taiwan." *Policy Options for Health Insurance and Long-Term Care Insurance*, ESRI Collaboration Projects (Macroeconomic Issues), March 2005. Last accessed August 15, 2016. http://www.esri.go.jp/jp/prj/int_prj/prj-2004_2005/macro/macro16/09-1-R.pdf.
Japan Center for International Exchange. 2006. "Building Effective Cross-Border and Regional Cooperation in East Asia." East Asian Regional Cooperation in the Fight Against HIV/AIDS, Tuberculosis, and Malaria (Beijing Conference 2006), 30–37. Tokyo: Japan Center for International Exchange.
J. W. Lee Center for Global Medicine. "Projects." Last accessed August 11, 2016. http://www.oldcgm.org/eng/globalm/projects/projects.php.
J. W. Lee Center for Global Medicine. 2014. "MOU: Lee Jong-wook geullobeol uihak denteo wa Laos bogeon daehakgyo gyoyuk kaebal senteo 2014.2.14 [MOU signed between J. W. Lee Center for Global Medicine and Educational Development Center, University of Health Sciences, Lao PDR, February 14, 2014]," February 15. Last accessed August 11, 2016. http://oldcgm.org/globalm/board/notice_view.php?key=&keyword=&bd_id=29.
Kang, Ae-ran. 2013. "Hwangol taltae dajim Seoul uidae uihak gyoyuk yeonguwon [Seoul National University College of Medicine's Planned Complete Overhaul of the NTTC]." *Daily medi*. September 4. Last accessed August 12, 2016. http://dailymedi.com/detail.php?number=771191.
Kang, Seong-man, Yang-jung Kim, and Yeong Hee Lee. 2012. "Gongjung bokeon ui daepok kamseo . . . Gyeongnam nong-eochon uiryo kongbaek uryeo [Large scale reduction in public health [services] . . . South Gyeongsang Province farming and fishing villages worried over the gaps in healthcare." *Yonhap News*: March 20, 2012. Last accessed August 15, 2016. http://www.yonhapnews.co.kr/bulletin/2012/03/20/0200000000AKR20120320025500052.HTML.

Kee, Chang Duk. 1996. "Joseon sidae mal kaemyeonggi ui uiryo (1) [Medicine during the Enlightenment Era of the Late Yi Dynasty (1)]." *Uihaksa [Korean Journal of Medical History]* 5 (2): 169–95.

———. 1996. "Joseon sidae mal kaemyeonggi ui uiryo (1) [Medicine during the Enlightenment Era of the Late Yi Dynasty (1)]." *Uihaksa [Korean Journal of Medical History]* 6 (1): 1–48.

Kim, Eun-yeong. 2014. "Gongbo-eui man barabogo innen jibang byeongweon deul." *Cheongnyeon uisa [Young Doctor]*, October 8. Last accessed August 15, 2016. http://www.docdocdoc.co.kr/161223.

Kim, Kyong-jee and Changwon Kee. 2012. "Reform of Medical Education in Korea." *Medical Teacher* 32: 113–17.

Kim, Kun-sang. 2004. "For Better Continuing Medical Education." *Journal of the Korean Medical Association* 47 (3): 184–87.

Kim, Kyong-jee, Joungho Han, Park le Byung, and Changwon Kee. 2009. "Medical Education in Korea: The e-learning Consortium." *Medical Teacher* 31 (9): e397–e401.

Kim, Ock Joo, and Sang Ik Hwang. 2000. "The Minnesota Project: The Influence of American Medicine on the Development of Medical Education and Medical Research in Post-War Korea." *Korean Journal of Medical History* 9 (1): 112–22.

Kim, Yeonjung, Chulsoo Lee, and Ilhak Lee. 2013. "Current Status and Prospects of Exchange of Health Officials from South and North Korea through Nongovernmental Organizations." *Journal of the Korean Medical Association* 56 (5): 375–82.

Korea Health and Development Institute. 2013. *The History of Medical Korea: from an International Medical Aid Recipient to a Donor*. New York: Korea Health and Development Institute.

Korean Association of Medical Education. 2010. "The Purpose of Establishment and History." KAMC Overview. Last accessed August 15, 2016. http://www.kamc.kr/eng/infor_02.html.

Korean Medical Association. "History." Last accessed August 15, 2016. http://www.kma.org/about/history.php.

Korean Medical Association. "Main Activities: The Measure of the Balance of Supply and Demand of Medical Human Resources and Development of Medical Education." Last accessed August 15, 2016. http://www.kma.org/english/7_activities.php?imagename=Image19&newimage=images/b_m7b.gif.

Lee, Eun-bin. 2013. "Konkukdae byeongwon, Zimbabwe eui simjang eul dasi ddwige hada [Konkuk University Hospital sets Zimbabwe's heart beating again]." *Uihyeop sinmun [Doctor's News]*, March 12. Last accessed August 15, 2016. http://www.doctorsnews.co.kr/news/articleView.html?idxno=94891.

Lee, Jong Chan, and Chang Duk Kee, 1996. "The Rise of Western Medicine and the Decline of Traditional Medicine in Korea, 1876–1910." *Korean Journal of Medical History* 5 (1): 1–9.

Lee, Wang-jun. 2006. "The Influence of Minnesota Project on the Korean Medical Education." PhD diss., Seoul National University. Cf. http://s-space.snu.ac.kr/handle/10371/19793.

Lee, Yoon-seong. 2008. "OSCE for the Medical Licensing Examination in Korea." *Kaohsiung Journal of Medical Science* 24 (12): 646–50.

Makoul, Gregory and Theo Schofield. 1999. "Communication Teaching and Assessment in Medical Education: An International Consensus Statement." *Patient Education and Counseling* 37 (1): 191–95.

Medical Service Act. 2011. Law No. 10609. (Republic of Korea.) Last accessed August 15, 2016. http://elaw.klri.re.kr/kor_service/lawView.do?hseq=29104&lang=ENG.

Newsis Press Service. 2012. "Kim Seon-yeong gyosu, Uganda e uidae chujin [Professor Kim Seon-yeong, Pushing for a Medical College in Uganda]," *Hankyoreh sinmun*, Society Section, April 22. Last accessed August 15, 2016. http://www.hani.co.kr/arti/society/health/529427.html.

Norris, Laurie. 2003. *The China Medical Board: 50 Years of Programs, Partnerships, and Progress, 1950–2000*. New York: China Medical Board of New York.

OECD/DAC Review Team. 2008. *DAC Special Review: Development Co-Operation of the Republic of Korea*. Paris: OECD Development Co-Operation Directorate. Last accessed August 15, 2016. http://www.oecd.org/dac/peer-reviews/42347329.pdf.

Park, Hoon-Ki. 2012. "The Impact of Introducing the Korean Medical Licensing Examination Clinical Skills Assessment on Medical Education." *Journal of the Korean Medical Association* 55 (2): 116–23.

Park, Yun-jae. 2004. "Reformation of the Medical Education Institutes and Training of General Doctors during the Early Period of Japanese Rule." *Journal of Korean Medical History* 13 (1): 20–36.

Seoul daehakgyo byeongwon byeongwon yoksa munhwa senteo [Seoul National University Hospital History and Culture Center]. 2009. *Sajin gwa hamkke bonun Hanguk keunhyeondae uiryo munhwasa 1876–1960 [A Pictorial History of Contemporary Korean Medical Culture, 1879–1960]*. Seoul: Woongjin ThinkBig.

Steger, Byron L. 1953. "Rehabilitation of Medical Education in South Korea." *United States Armed Forces Medical Journal* 4 (12): 1675–92.

Stoddard, G. D. 1959. "Report of ICA Consultant on Higher Education in Korea with Special Reference to Seoul National University and the Contracts between ICA and US Universities." Unpublished report, International Cooperation Agency, Washington, DC.

Tagore, Rabindranath. 2006. "Lamp of the East." In *East Asian Literatures: An Interface with India*, edited by P. A. George, 97. New Delhi: Northern Book Centre.

Yeo, In-sok, Hyun-sook Lee, Seong-su Kim, Gyu-hwan Sin, Yun-hyeong Park, and Yun-jae Park. 2012. *Hanguk Uihaksa [History of Korean Medicine]*. Seoul: Daehan uisa hyeophoe Uiryo jeongchaek yeonguso [Research Institute for Healthcare Policy, Korean Medical Association].

Yonsei University Health System. 2009. "College of Medicine." Last accessed November 7, 2015. http://www.yuhs.or.kr/en/Edu_Research/Coll_Medicine/.

Yoo, Seung Yoon. 2006. "Survey of CME Recognition and Satisfaction among Primary Care Physicians." *Journal of Korean Medical Education* 18 (1): 85–93.

part III
Future Challenges

8 Burden of Disease: Implications for Medical Education in East Asia

Stuart Gilmour, Yusuke Tsugawa, and Kenji Shibuya

Introduction

In 1914, when John Rockefeller created the China Medical Board (CMB), Chinese life expectancy was a mere thirty-five years (Chen and Ling 2014). East Asian countries were suffering from poverty, famine, and communicable diseases. A hundred years later, these countries have experienced major socioeconomic development, starting with Japan in the late 1950s, South Korea in the 1980s, and China in the 1990s. These countries now face rapid aging and have reached the current stage of epidemiological transition with a growing burden of noncommunicable diseases (NCDs) (Khang 2013; G. Yang et al. 2013). They share similar historical and cultural backgrounds, but they also have stark differences in their political, economic, and institutional arrangements.

East Asia is probably one of the most dynamic and interconnected regions of the world, and it is becoming the focus of the global health community in the twenty-first century. Understanding the commonalities and differences in population health in this region is critical for the future of not only national health systems but also of the global health community. Although the national health systems of these countries have been compared in terms of health financing (Wagstaff 2005), and although individual countries in the region have all been described in terms of burden of disease (G. Yang et al. 2013), risk factors (Ikeda et al. 2012), and health systems challenges (Shibuya 2011a; Shibuya et al. 2011b), a comprehensive comparison on the basis of burden of disease, with attention to the lessons that can be learned globally from their experiences and challenges, has not yet been conducted. This chapter provides an overview of the comparative analysis of disease burden and risk factors in three East Asian countries (China, Japan, and South Korea). The chapter concludes with a discussion of the future of national health systems in an aging and interconnected world and the implications of the Global Burden of Disease (GBD) analysis for medical education in East Asia, emphasizing contributions to global health.

Burden of Disease in East Asia

The GBD study is a systematic scientific effort to quantify the comparative magnitude of health loss due to diseases, injuries, and risk factors by age, sex, and geographies for specific points in time (Murray et al. 2012a), and it enables the calculation of consistent and comparable measures of health loss from diseases and injuries (Murray et al. 2012b) and the assessment of associated risk factors (Lim et al. 2012). The study integrates death and disability, enabling countries to compare the effect of different diseases, injuries, and risk factors in order to set health policy based on objective and comparable information (Murray et al. 2013). The GBD 2010 revision was a continuation of work initiated by the World Bank, World Health Organization, and Harvard University in 1991 and systematically assessed all the available evidence on mortality and morbidity from 291 causes and 55 risk factors, as well as 1,163 disease and injury sequelae. GBD 2010 was a completely new analysis using new methods to obtain revised results for 187 countries and 21 regions in 1990, 2005, and 2010, with uncertainty intervals for all quantities of interest. Results from the GBD project, which is now regularly updated, provide important mechanisms and tools for understanding the diseases and risk factors that countries should focus on in order to improve population health (Horton 2010). In this section, we review the patterns of disease and mortality in three East Asian countries and the implications for their national health policies.

Substantial Declines in Rapid Aging and Mortality

Amartya Sen once suggested using mortality, instead of gross national income, as an index of success or failure of economic development (Sen 1995). It is obvious that one of the greatest achievements in the twentieth century was the substantial decline in both child and adult mortality, resulting in a huge increase in average life expectancy at birth across the world. The most dramatic and rapid gains in population health have occurred in East Asia, where life expectancy at birth increased from less than forty-five years in 1950 to more than seventy-four years today (United Nations Population Division 2012).

Immediately after World War II, the health status of the Japanese population was poor: male life expectancy at birth was only fifty years and female life expectancy only fifty-four years (ibid.). But since then, Japan has ranked first in terms of female life expectancy at birth since 1986 and has continued to reduce adult mortality among those aged sixty to eighty years old (Lozano et al. 2012). From 1990 to 2010, female and male life expectancy at birth in Japan also increased, from 81.9 to 86.4 years and from 75.9 to 79.6 years, respectively. However, the pace of decline in adult mortality has been slower than some other nations in recent years, and it is possible that, if recent trends continue, other nations are likely to achieve lower rates of adult mortality than Japan (Murray 2011).

China and South Korea have made huge health gains in the past twenty years, and at a much faster pace than those Japan experienced during the 1960s–1980s. One of the major achievements in global health is China's performance in Millennium Development Goals (MDGs) related to maternal, newborn, and child health, as well as in decreasing the prevalence of tuberculosis (G. Yang et al. 2013). There has also been a large decline in mortality in all age groups (approximately 45 percent reduction on average), and the greatest reductions were in female children aged one to four years (71 percent) (Lozano et al. 2012). In South Korea, age-specific all-cause mortality rates have shown significant declines from 1990 to 2010 in every age group, with the largest reductions in children aged one to five years (ibid.; S. Yang et al. 2010). There have also been very rapid reductions in female adult mortality (S. Yang et al. 2012), with the smallest reduction being found among those over eighty years of age.

Advanced Health Transitions

The six figures show the findings from the 2013 GBD study for the years 1990 and 2010 for age- and cause-specific burden of disease in China (figs. 8.1A–B, respectively 1990 and 2010), Japan (figs. 8.2A–B), and South Korea (figs. 8.3A–B). These stacked bar charts show disability-adjusted life years (DALYs) by five-year age category for each country. Each bar is subdivided by major categories of disease type, color-coded for easy reference. The burden of disease here is quantified in absolute numbers in order to show the total magnitude of disease burden as it has changed over time. The three countries share some disease burden and risk factor profiles specific to East Asia (e.g., stroke, infection-related cancers, smoking, and high blood pressure), but there are also significant differences across the countries, particularly in the distribution of burden among age groups and the relative importance of cardiovascular and cancer causes among older age groups.

China has successfully reduced its disease burden from maternal, newborn, and child causes, and tuberculosis, which resulted in a rapid health transition with an increasing burden from noncommunicable disease and injuries (*The Lancet* Editors 2013). This shift in burden corresponds to a decline in the influence of infectious diseases more generally, consistent with the nation's shift into the epidemiological patterns found in more developed countries. In particular, childhood pneumonia showed the largest change in contribution to health burden, falling by 80 percent from 1990 to 2010, and stroke, ischemic heart disease, chronic obstructive pulmonary disease, road injuries, and lung cancer were the leading causes of disease burden in 2010 (G. Yang et al. 2013). Other noncommunicable diseases associated with this health transition have also grown in significance: renal diseases and diabetes, for example, have grown in magnitude over the past twenty years, while the burden of cancer in younger age groups has grown as well.

This changed epidemiological pattern is also apparent in Figure 8.4, which shows the ranking of the top twenty-five causes of burden of disease in China compared to three other East Asian countries. Liver cancer, primarily due to hepatitis infection, is still among the top ten causes of disease in China and was ranked tenth in 2010, but other infectious diseases did not rank in the top ten. Despite a lower prevalence of disabilities when compared with other countries, there is a growing burden from disabling conditions due to lower back pain, major depressive disorder, neck pain, other musculo-skeletal disorders, and diabetes. The progress of China and South Korea through the epidemiological transition is apparent in Figure 8.4, where some causes that remain highly ranked in these two countries have a much lower presence in Japan, indicating that China and South Korea are yet to complete the epidemiological transition completely.

There is not much difference between the highest ranked causes of disease burden in Japan in 1990 and those in 2010. The leading causes of DALYs in 2010 were lower back pain, stroke, ischemic heart disease, pneumonia, and other musculo-skeletal disorders, while suicide was still an important cause of health loss. In South Korea, the health transition has further accelerated during the past two decades. Stroke, suicide, ischemic heart disease, liver cancer, and stomach cancer were the top five leading causes of DALYs. The causes that were in the ten leading causes of DALYs in 2010 but not in 1990 were suicide, other musculo-skeletal disorders, and neck pain. And so, a growing burden from disabling non-communicable conditions is apparent, including lower back pain, neck pain, other musculo-skeletal disorders, major depressive disorder, and anxiety disorders.

A Comparative Analysis of Risk Factors

Figure 8.5 shows the comparative assessment of disease burden attributable to major risk factors for China, Japan, and South Korea. In these three countries, dietary risks were the leading risk factor and both high blood pressure and smoking were consistently among the top five risk factors. Air pollution and alcohol use are exceptionally high in China and South Korea, whereas Japan experienced increased prevalence of obesity and physical inactivity among the top ten risk factors.

While South Korea faces a similar disease burden to Japan as it moves forward with its epidemiological transition, the GBD 2013 identifies a different set of health challenges for China. Although China's transition is well underway, there is still a heavy burden of stroke, as well as environmental and infectious disease risk factors. Both Japan and South Korea could provide opportunities and lessons for the Chinese health system to act quickly and effectively against major NCDs and their risk factors.

For example, rapid health gains in Japan during the 1960s–1980s could be attributable not only to socioeconomic development but also to the implementation

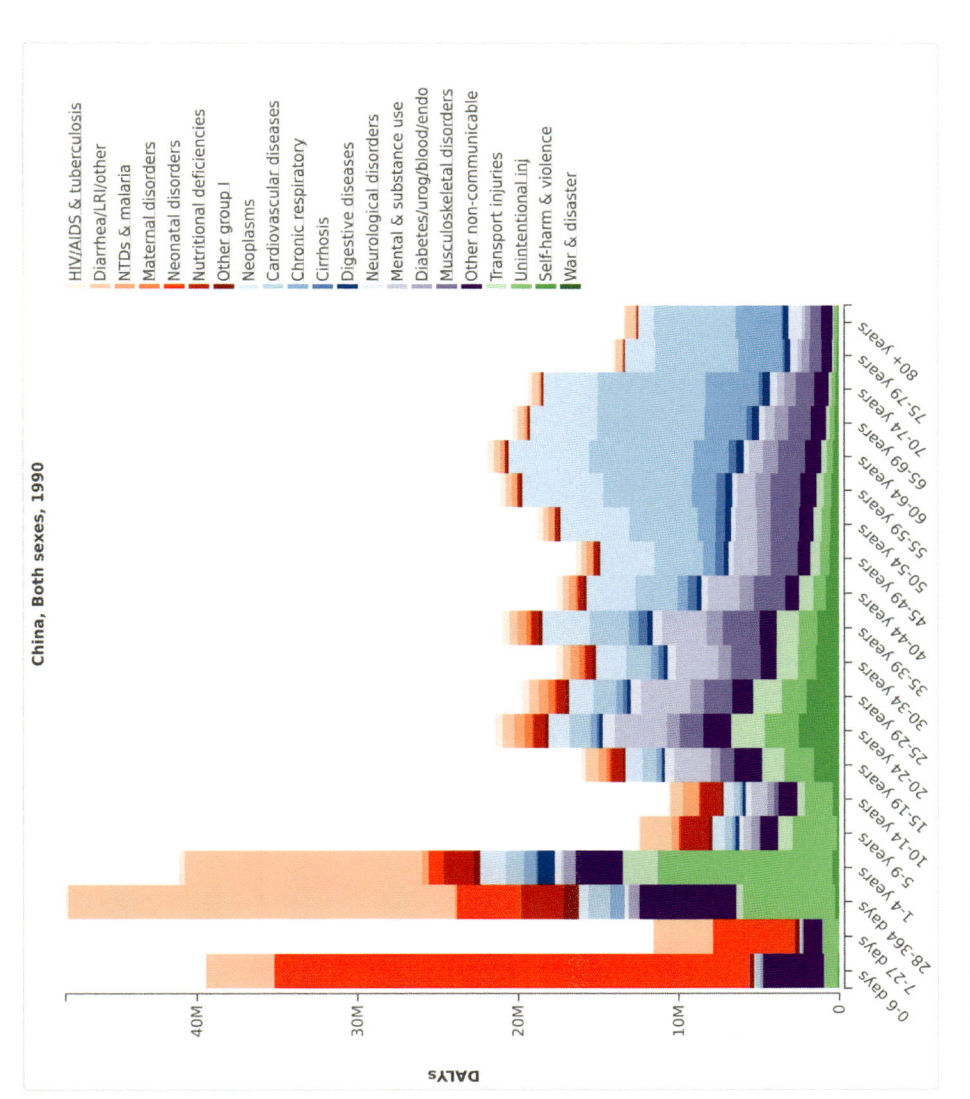

Fig. 8.1A Burden of Disease in China in 1990.

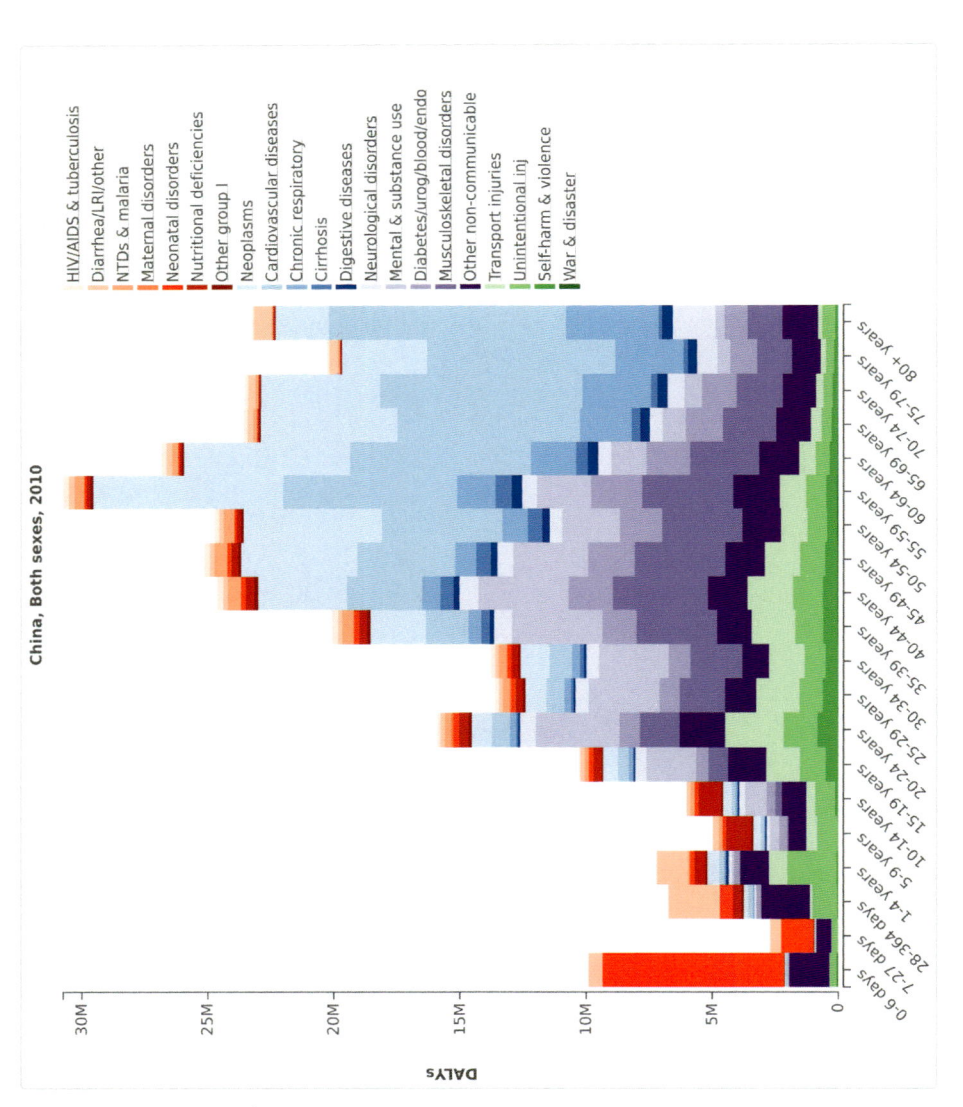

Fig. 8.1B Burden of Disease in China in 2010.

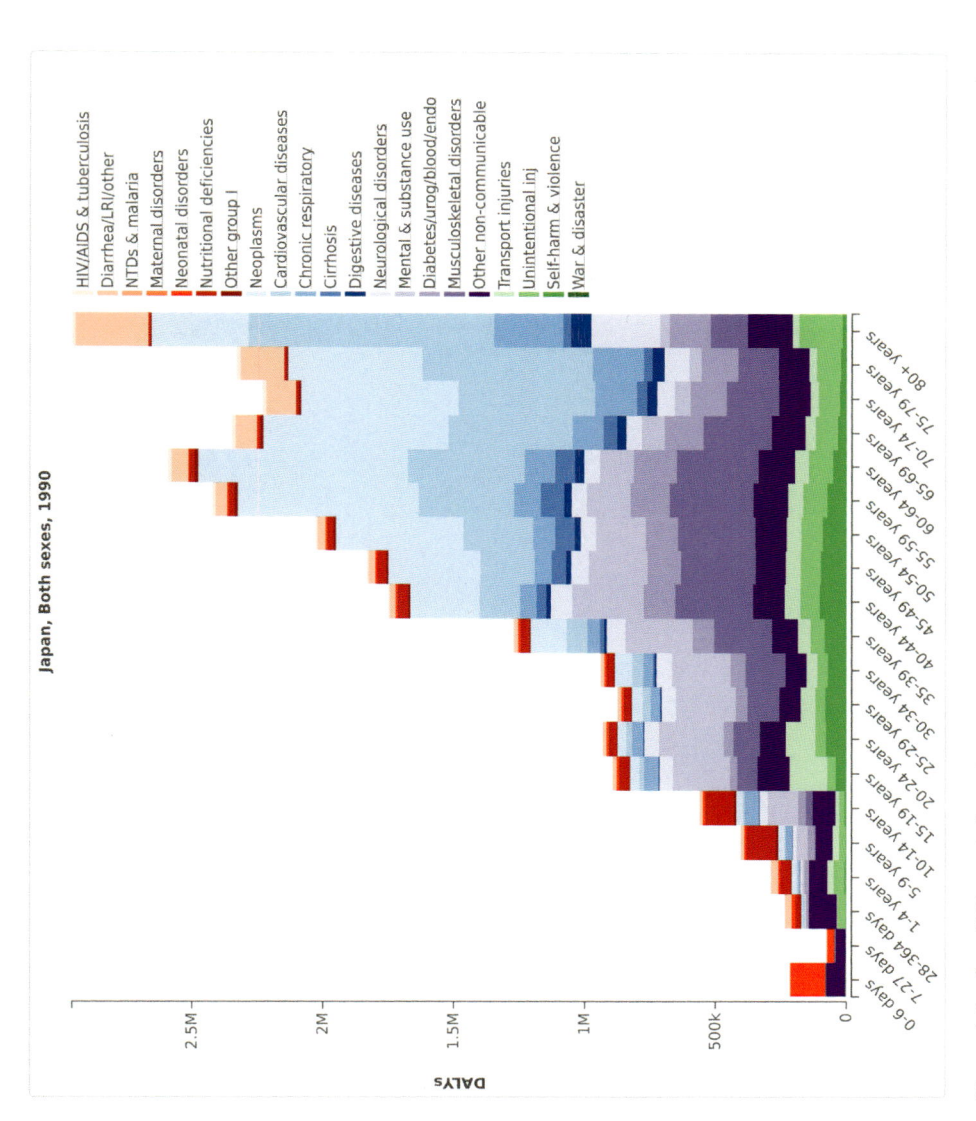

Fig. 8.2A Burden of Disease in Japan in 1990.

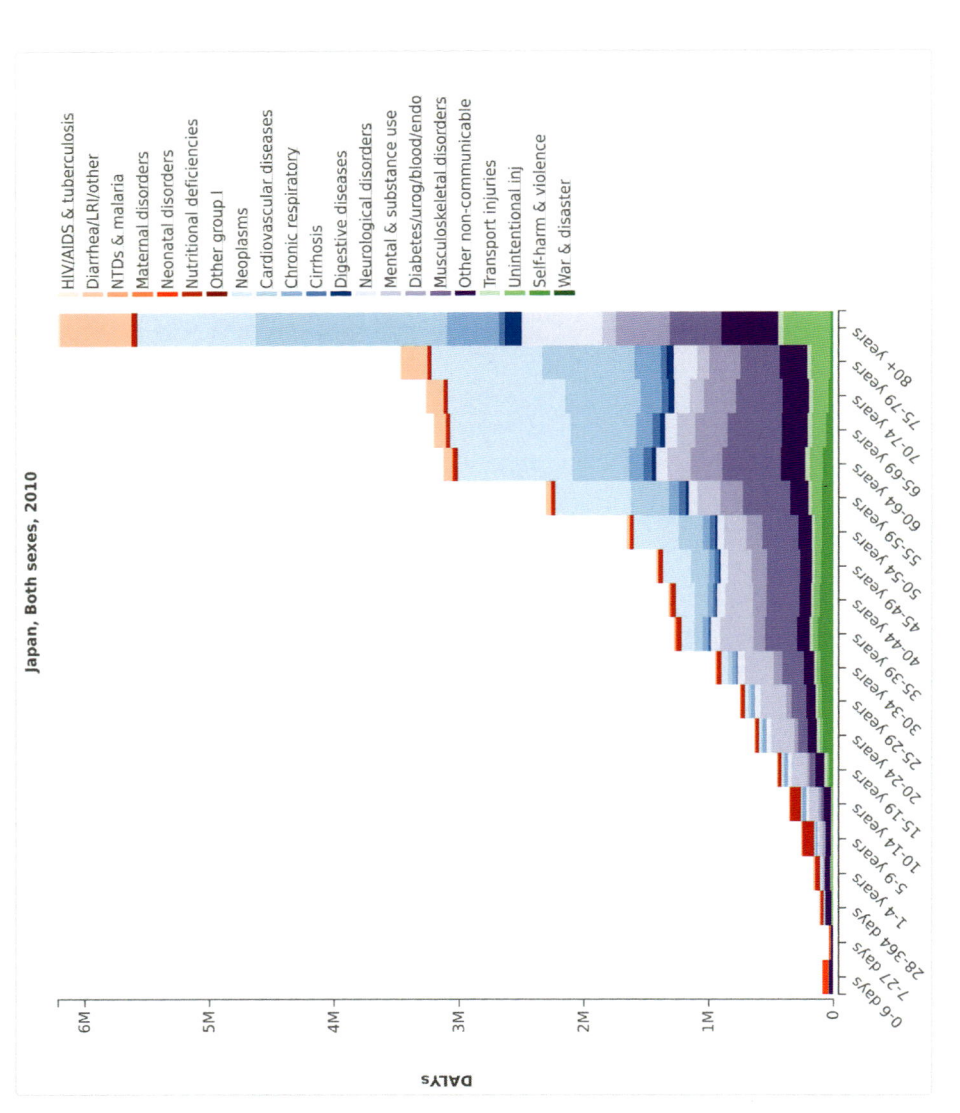

Fig. 8.2B Burden of Disease in Japan in 2010.

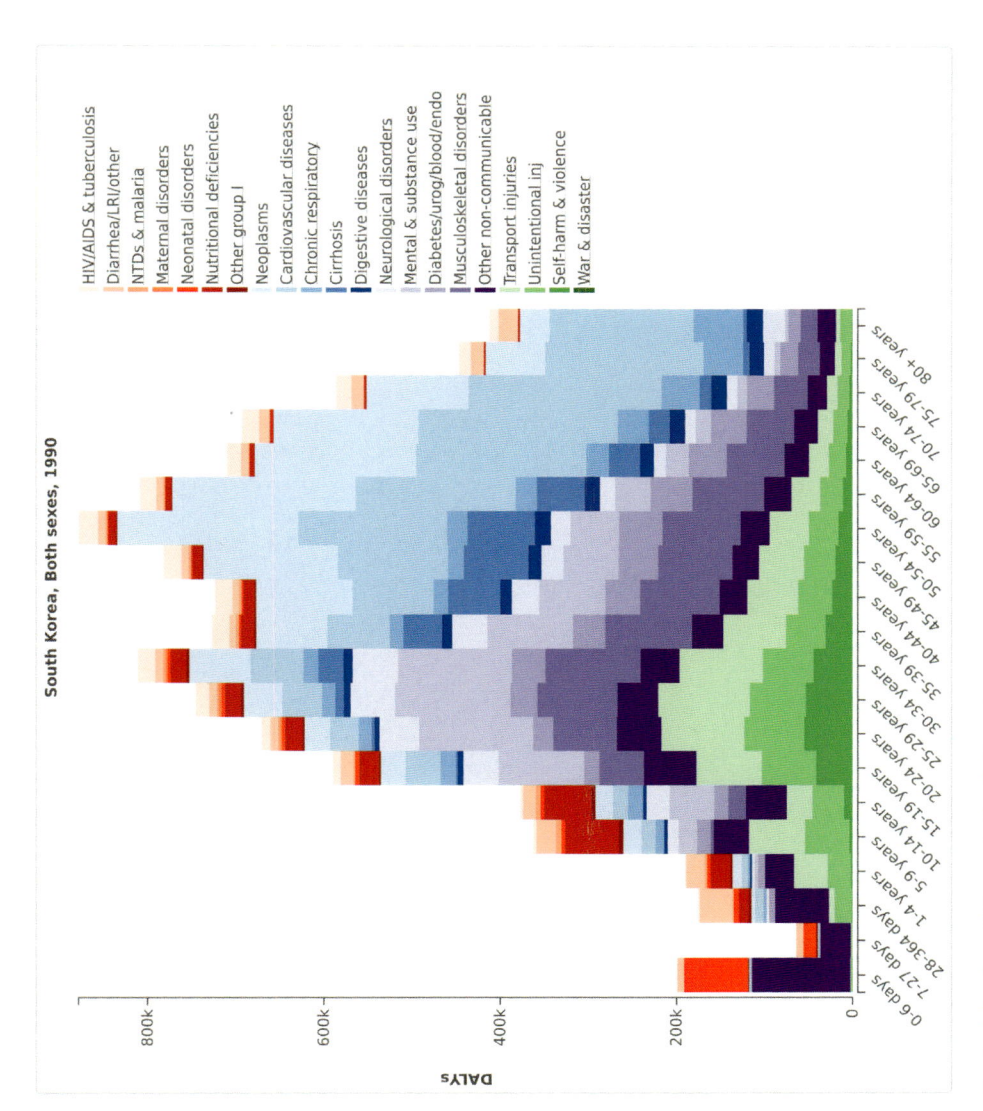

Fig. 8.3A Burden of Disease in South Korea in 1990.

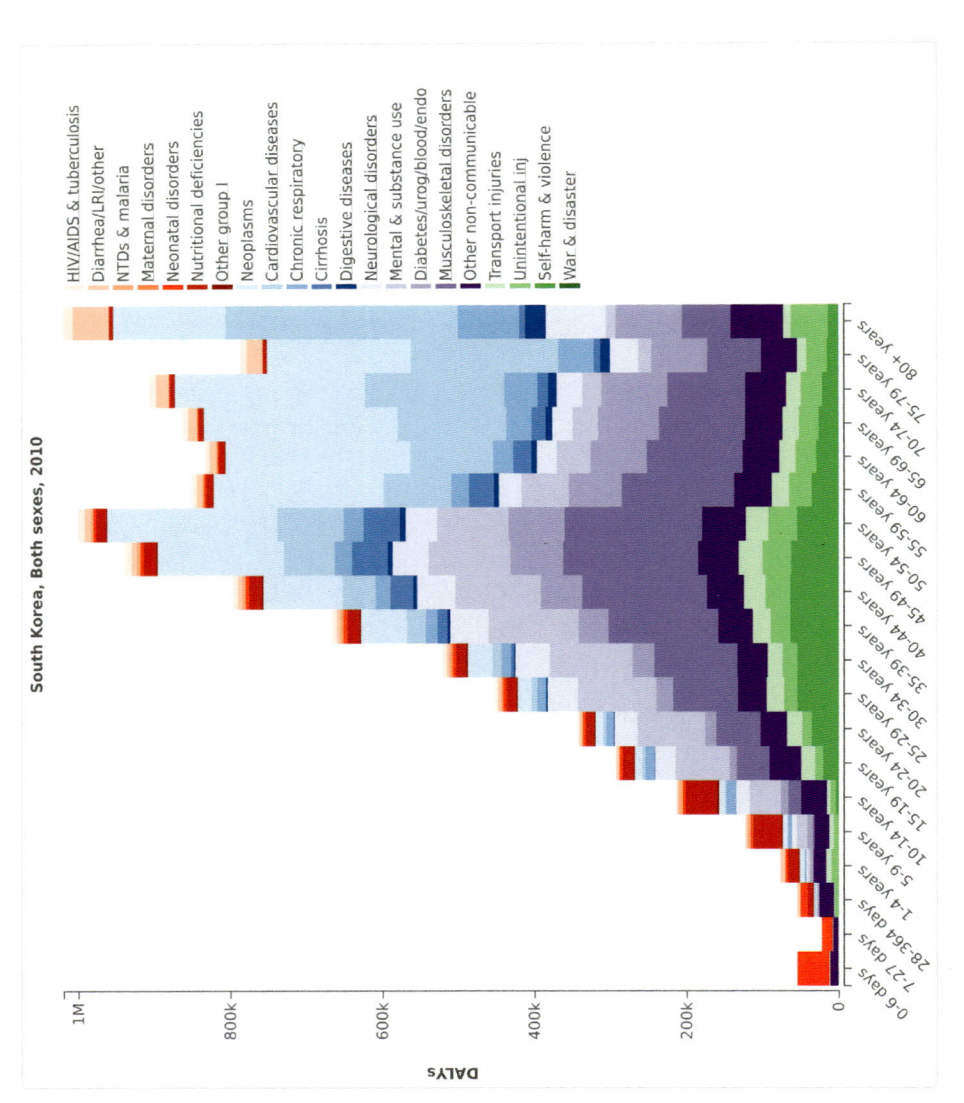

Fig. 8.3B Burden of Disease in South Korea in 2010.

Both sexes, All ages, 2010, DALYs

	China	Japan	S Korea
Cerebrovascular disease	1	2	2
Low back & neck pain	2	1	1
Ischemic heart disease	3	3	5
Road injuries	4	25	12
COPD	5	12	16
Lung cancer	6	5	7
Depressive disorders	7	8	13
Sense organ diseases	8	11	14
Diabetes	9	10	4
Liver cancer	10	16	6
Skin diseases	11	13	11
Stomach cancer	12	9	8
Congenital anomalies	13	29	29
Neonatal preterm birth	14	60	42
Lower respiratory infect	15	4	24
Schizophrenia	16	30	23
Other musculoskeletal	17	6	9
Self-harm	18	7	3
Iron-deficiency anemia	19	19	15
Falls	20	17	17
Chronic kidney disease	21	18	20
Drowning	22	55	49
Esophageal cancer	23	37	51
Neonatal encephalopathy	24	95	79
Anxiety disorders	25	31	19

Fig. 8.4 Rankings of Burden of Disease in East Asia in 2010.

Both sexes, All ages, 2010, DALYs

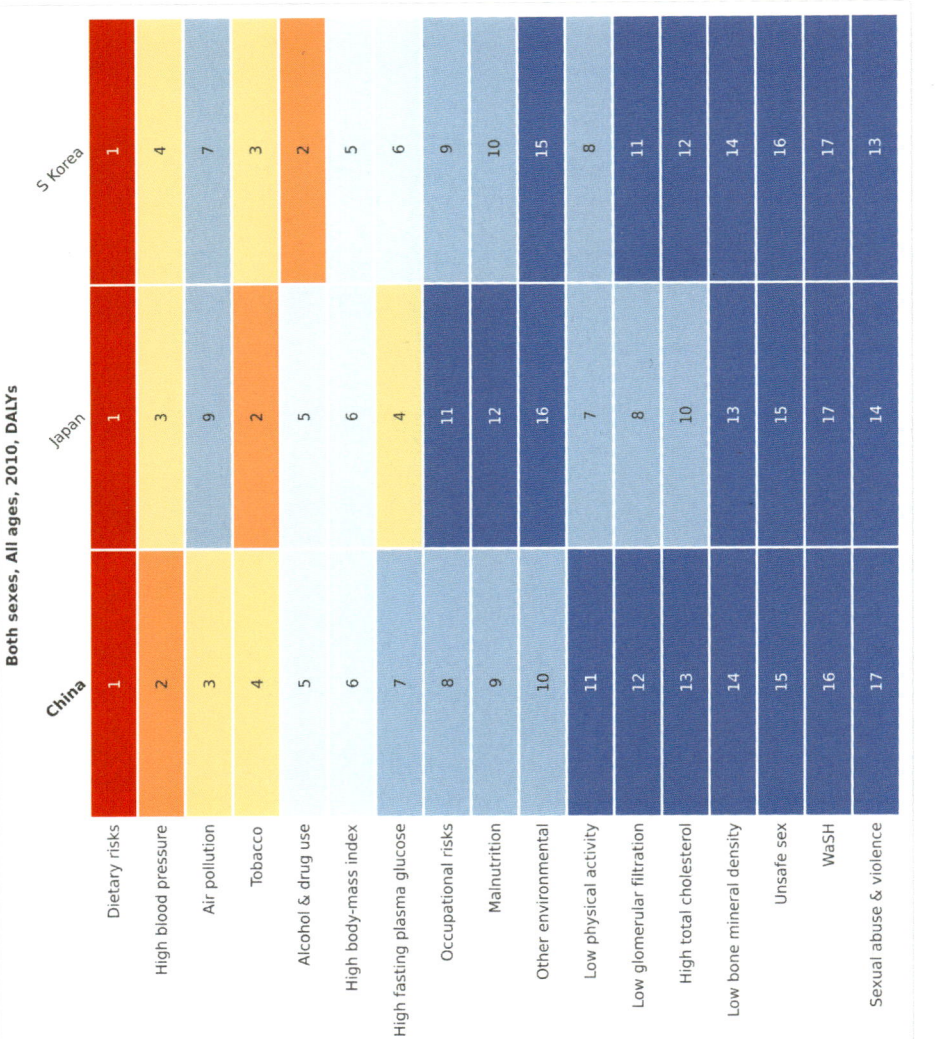

	China	Japan	S Korea
Dietary risks	1	1	1
High blood pressure	2	3	4
Air pollution	3	9	7
Tobacco	4	2	3
Alcohol & drug use	5	5	2
High body-mass index	6	6	5
High fasting plasma glucose	7	4	6
Occupational risks	8	11	9
Malnutrition	9	12	10
Other environmental	10	16	15
Low physical activity	11	7	8
Low glomerular filtration	12	8	11
High total cholesterol	13	10	12
Low bone mineral density	14	13	14
Unsafe sex	15	15	16
WaSH	16	17	17
Sexual abuse & violence	17	14	13

Fig. 8.5 Rankings of Risk Factors in East Asia in 2010.

of primary and secondary preventive community public health measures against noncommunicable diseases, such as salt reduction campaigns and air pollution legislation, as well as an increased use of advanced medical technologies, such as antihypertensive agents, through the universal insurance scheme (Ikeda et al. 2012; Roth et al. 2011). Since then, Japan has imposed a series of interventions, including strict air pollution control legislation and the development of clean air technologies that have reduced the large disease, financial, and social burden due to PM (particulate matter) air pollution, a problem still noticeable in China's burden of disease statistics.

On the other hand, the pace of mortality decline for adults in Japan has been slower than some other nations in recent years. Such stagnation is related partly to high tobacco consumption, high suicide rates, and other risk factors. For example, the combined prevalence of overweight and obesity has increased from 21 percent to 25 percent there since 1990 (Ng et al. 2014), and tobacco use has declined slowly over this period relative to other high-income countries (Bilano et al. 2015). Progress in the management of chronic illness has also been slow, partly due to the poor quality of primary care (Lim et al. 2012; Murray et al. 2013). Only half of patients currently receiving drugs to control high blood pressure and hypercholesterolemia achieved targeted levels of outcomes in Japan (Ikeda et al. 2012). Moreover, the number of undiagnosed and untreated patients in the community was greater than the estimated numbers from the 2007 US National Health and Nutrition Examination Survey (Hashimoto et al. 2011).

Sub-National Burden of Disease Estimation and Policy Development

China, Japan, and South Korea have all started their own national and subnational burden of disease analysis, funded by national ministries of health. These studies enable national policymakers to answer important questions about geographical variation in the burden of disease within their countries, the relative importance of inequality in determining disease burden, and important occupational risks (Gilmour et al. 2014). They also provide detailed information about region-specific and urban-rural divides in the burden of disease, which is often sought by local authorities for health system planning. Provision of such information enables better collaboration between local health authorities, better coordination of national plans, and a better understanding of past achievements and future health risks.

Similarly, the GBD studies can be used as the basis for comparative health assessment internationally, enabling health outcomes between countries with diverse social and health systems to be compared in a consistent and rigorous manner (Institute for Health Metrics and Evaluation 2013). The GBD approach, with its focus on comparability, consistency, and comprehensiveness of disease and risk factor analysis between countries, makes it a useful tool to implement comparative health system assessment, to design public health programs and preventive interventions (Kim 2012), and to identify gaps in international data systems (Chan 2012). Although problems remain in comparing even geographically close and culturally similar countries (due to different local definitions of exposures, differing approaches to life expectancy, and challenges of data comparability), the GBD approach remains the most comprehensive and consistent method for cross-national comparisons.

The GBD 2010 study was initiated in 2007 with a grant from the Bill and Melinda Gates Foundation. The Institute of Health Metrics and Evaluation at the University of Washington in Seattle is a coordinating institution in collaboration with partner institutions including the University of Queensland, WHO, Harvard University, Johns Hopkins University, Imperial College, and the University of Tokyo. Over 450 authors signed up for the GBD 2010 series in *The Lancet* (Institute for Health Metrics and Evaluation 2012). However, the current GBD process is essentially a unilateral process (GBD 1.0) in which academics publish the results in paper publications or on websites. In order for the GBD process to be truly collaborative and enhance a joint learning process (GBD 2.0), among three East Asia countries that are working on the national and sub-national burden of disease analysis independently, for example, the GBD process needs to expand across a network of country-population health experts and strengthen core analytical capacities. East Asian countries have the national capacity to facilitate such a process. By incorporating national-level collaborators and more detailed data, it is hoped that even more accurate estimates can be produced and updated frequently.

The Future of Health Policy in East Asia

Our analysis of the burden of disease shows three key factors that are shaping the population health profiles in East Asia: rapid aging, increasing disabilities due to the NCDs epidemic, and an unfinished agenda of controlling infectious diseases. Rapid aging drives a shift in the burden of disease away from easily preventable illnesses of childhood and toward complex, interrelated diseases that occur over the course of life, requiring a shift away from strictly clinical, specialist medical functions and toward integrated health services. The growth of NCDs and their entrenched risk factors, such as obesity and tobacco use, leads to an increasing burden of disability, driving the focus of health systems away from the treatment of acute symptoms in classical clinical settings to community care for disease management and rehabilitation. Despite this transition to a higher prevalence of NCDs, the unfinished agenda of controlling infectious diseases requires continued attention both to preventable childhood diseases that threaten to return in high-income countries (e.g., rubella) and to some categories of infectious disease that have not yet been fully managed, especially lower respiratory tract infections. Together with a growing sense of inequity—in terms of both economics and health (Ikegami et al. 2011)—these factors are imposing a substantial burden on national and regional health systems, one for which present personnel in those systems are not yet fully prepared.

These changes in the burden of disease and in the challenges that East Asia faces require both a new global health paradigm and radical changes in the way that the health workforce is educated and deployed. In this section, we describe this new global health paradigm and its relation to the health challenges in East Asia. We outline the reforms in medical education that are needed to properly prepare the medical workforce for the world after this epidemiological transition, where smart use of data and integrated health systems within a new network of international and national organizations will lead to revolutionary new forms of health care practice.

A New Global Health Paradigm

The response to these challenges among health systems in East Asia is confounded by three broader trends in the health sector that arise from changes in the ways the modern world uses and disseminates information and integrates its different sectors. The future of the health sector lies in recognition of major shifts in information management, its integration within and across a wider sector that is larger than just the traditional health sector, and its need to respond to the globalization of health risks and responsibilities. Like other sectors, the health sector is no longer isolated, and it needs to learn to adapt to an interconnected world.

Through better use of the most revolutionary information management ideas, the health sector is finding new and intelligent ways to access, share, and utilize information. This means looking beyond the traditional keystones of vital registration and hospital data, toward incorporating the distributed information available through the internet and personal communications devices and leveraging data-sharing opportunities across the health care and social care sector. It also means merging data and sharing knowledge outside of the traditional health sector, and nowhere is this clearer than in the wider life sciences sector.

Here, access to unique genetic data and information from the wider biosciences and allied health community will enable unique new techniques for drug targeting and more intelligent interventions (Burke et al. 2006), which are particularly important in dealing with complex, multifaceted risk factors that are common to the NCD epidemic. Finally, as the health profile of East Asian nations converges, the risks that they share begin to cross national boundaries within and beyond this region: changes in diet and physical activity patterns, environmental risk factors such as air pollution and global warming that are shared across the region, and migration all serve to globalize risk beyond the traditional paradigm of infectious diseases (Woodward et al. 2011; Beaglehole and Yach 2003). For such complex interrelated risk factors driven by environmental and global trends in lifestyle and markets, information alone will not be sufficient to change individual behaviors, and increased attention to social and environmental determinants of health will be needed. But without quality data and a health workforce trained to understand, use, and deploy knowledge, the health sector will not be ready for this challenge.

In the same way that changes in the information management sector offer many lessons to health care, so can other sectors. Just as the retail industry has transformed in a few decades from small shops to huge, distributed delivery systems like Walmart and Amazon, so also the health sector must move to create larger, networked, and integrated systems of care with a greater focus on clearer standards and quality (Cutler 2013). From individual clinics to group practices, efficiency and effectiveness can be improved by integrating care in larger systems and networks. These may not be physically colocated, but the use of information management tools to coordinate and link these systems will enable them to do everything that is needed over the life of a patient: health checks, treatment of acute disease such as heart failure, nursing and social care for the elderly, and routine management of risk factors and chronic illness.

However, a traditional and paternalistic approach to public health through information provision alone will not substantially improve health behaviors and outcomes at the individual level (World Health Organization 2010; Marmot 2005). There has been growing evidence on the relevance of social and environmental determinants of health at both national and global levels and on the need for inter-sectoral action to address them (Marmot 2013; World Health Organization 1986). Recent policy innovations by the Japanese Ministry of Health, Labour, and Welfare recognize this, leading to the development of a new program of community-based integrated care that links health care, long-term care, prevention, and livelihood support at the community level, ensuring that the complex health challenges associated with an aging population are managed through a coordinated response. This paradigm uses networked information and integrated services to provide standardized care focusing on outcomes that can be measured in real time and aims to improve standards of care while reducing costs. It will also involve patients, their families, and their communities in care, recognizing that health practitioners and patients have changing roles in an interconnected society (Cutler 2011). This paradigm was formalized in 2015 with the publication of Health Care 2035, the report of an official advisory panel to the Health Minister of Japan that incorporated these concepts of community and personal engagement, fairness, and solidarity in a vision for the country's health system during a period of rapid aging (Miyata et al. 2015).

Recognizing this integrated and interconnected society and its effect on health is an essential part of this new vision for health care as going far beyond the traditional heath sectors and national boundaries. In an increasingly interdependent modern society with changing relations between the young and the elderly, men and women, and doctors and patients, people cannot live in isolation, and the social context of health is an important component of the system. Experience in rebuilding from the Great East Japan Earthquake and Tsunami has shown the importance of this connectedness in securing health: temporary housing for evacuees that isolates them from their community makes it impossible to improve their health, and as a result, the Mayor of Soma City has introduced terraced houses and community workers to ensure that the community can work together and share in the support of its own health (Tachiya 2011). This has wider lessons for aging societies, which need to find new ways to rebuild communities and human relationships and new ways of thinking about aging and health. But this cannot be done without changes in the way medical professionals view health and health systems and their social context.

Reforming Medical Education for the Twenty-First Century

The challenges facing East Asian countries in terms of population aging, NCD burden, and the changing global health paradigm require a new approach to medical practice, a shift away from an emphasis on specialist practitioners working to treat symptoms in a clinical setting and toward integrated health teams with a primary health care and prevention focus that coordinate with workers outside of the traditional health sector and incorporate intelligent use and understanding of data so as to comprehend their patients' health in the context of a life course of accrued NCD risk and long-term care. The traditional medical education system is not prepared for this radical shift in approach to health (Jason and Douglas 2015). These shortcomings of traditional medical education are no less acute in East Asia, where medical education systems have been modeled on the systems developed from the 1910 Flexner report (Bullock 2011), but where aging and the health transition will bring these challenges into focus most rapidly.

Historically, medical education has been focused on the needs of those who provide the education, rather than the interests of the broader community that students will ultimately serve. Medical curriculums are centered around practical, common sense approaches to historically important illnesses and are often delivered by university professors who are well-respected in their field and have strong and specific views on the issues they teach. Departments, department chairs, and medical organizations have a great deal of authority over what is taught, and in combination, these elements generate an inertia that makes it difficult to change curriculums to make them more responsive to their students and the community.

However, change is necessary if the medical profession is to keep pace with rapid population aging, the epidemiological transition, and the coming shifts in information, integration, and globalization, especially in East Asia. Medical education needs to reflect the needs of those who will use these services in the future and to consider the demand-side pressures on health services. These pressures can arise from the community, from government, and from global health organizations that need doctors to be capable of working in multidisciplinary settings and, increasingly, multinational contexts. To respond to these needs, a medical curriculum needs to include closer understanding of the population burden of disease through greater incorporation of burden of disease estimates into curriculum design. Moreover, the medical curriculum needs to incorporate understanding of the care value chain cycle (Porter and Teisberg 2006), rather than only respond to specific symptoms and narrow disease categories, in order to better integrate community care into the point of service. Finally, the medical curriculum needs to include awareness and appreciation of what the population expects from doctors and clinics. By moving beyond a narrow clinical point-of-care model and recognizing that health professionals are not the only way to address disease, medical education can begin to respond to the challenges of the interconnected, globalized world of modern epidemiology, particularly through the burden-of-disease approach.

The new paradigm for global health also requires health professionals who are trained in policy analysis, leadership, management, and communication with various stakeholders (Horton 2010). Health professionals with these capabilities will need to be educated under a new framework of both professional practice and personal development, which the Commission on Education of Health Professionals for the Twenty-First Century described as "transformative" (Ban and Fetters 2011). Given the rapid aging and advanced epidemiological transition in East Asia, which imposes a substantial burden on the sustainability of its future health systems, this bold and challenging paradigm for the future of health education has the potential to offer greater promise in East Asia than in other regions.

One example of this new educational model in action is the Global Leadership Program (GLP) at the University of Tokyo. GLP is unique compared to other programs offered by universities in Japan. The curriculum, taught entirely in English, offers elements drawn from the global forefront of knowledge, with both academic and field-based perspectives of a quality accessible to doctoral and postdoctoral students. GLP maintains a constant focus on the importance of practical interventions and policy development informed by data through seminars and workshops in which analysis and data synthesis are integrated in all discussions. The results of the GBD are given a key place in this process, and students leave GLP well-versed in the use of data to inform policy, understanding the importance of the disease context as a part of objective decision-making. Along with similar efforts at the Global Health Unit at the Peking University Health Science Center and J. W. Lee Center at Seoul National University, GLP is an example of a model of education reform intended to prepare medical graduates for the health challenges of the twenty-first century.

Conclusion

The Global Burden of Disease (GBD) study shows the pace at which health has changed in East Asia in just over a century. From nations struggling with poverty, famine, and infectious diseases, East Asian nations have grown to become developed industrial powerhouses facing complex and interconnected health problems in an increasingly globalized world. The GBD also shows the value of global information and shared knowledge for understanding and responding to new health challenges. Comparative analysis between countries with similar growth and development trajectories but with very different current health concerns enables all the nations in East Asia to learn from each other's experience, to share knowledge, and to collaborate in achieving key global health goals.

But the new health challenges represented by the GBD are not necessarily reflected in medical education, and a new paradigm in medical education is needed to enable the health workforce to adapt to a new global health model built on information sharing, partnership, and leadership. Medical education both inside and outside of East Asia needs to adapt to this new global paradigm in health if the remarkable health gains of the past hundred years are to continue into the twenty-first century.

Furthermore, as part of the global community, the nations of East Asia have an opportunity and responsibility to share their experience of rapid health gains, managing the epidemiological transition, and adapting to population aging with those countries in the rest of the world that will soon follow the same path of increased prevalence of aging populations, noncommunicable diseases, and complex behavioral and health problems. This process of sharing and learning will depend on health professionals educated to interact with global health systems and will require education systems to adapt to make this possible. At the University of Tokyo and elsewhere, this process has begun, but larger steps are needed both across and beyond academia if the lessons of health improvement in East Asia are to be continued and the benefit spread throughout the whole world.

References

Ban, Nobutaro, and Michael D. Fetters. 2011. "Education for Health Professionals in Japan—Time to Change." *The Lancet* 378 (9798): 1206–07.

Beaglehole, Robert, and Derek Yach. 2003. "Globalisation and the Prevention and Control of Non-Communicable Disease: The Neglected Chronic Diseases of Adults." *The Lancet* 362 (9387): 903–08.

Bilano, Ver, Stuart Gilmour, Trevor Moffiet, Edouard Tursan d'Espaignet, Gretchen A. Stevens, Alison Commar, Frank Tuyl, et al. 2015. "Global Trends and Projections for Tobacco Use, 1990–2025: An Analysis of Smoking Indicators from the WHO Comprehensive Information Systems for Tobacco Control." *The Lancet* 385 (9972): 966–76.

Bullock, Mary Brown. 2011. *The Oil Prince's Legacy: Rockefeller Philanthropy in China*. Washington, DC: Woodrow Wilson Center and Stanford University Press.

Burke, Wylie, Muin J. Khoury, Alison Stewart, and Ronald L. Zimmern for the Bellagio Group. 2006. "The Path from Genome-Based Research to Population Health: Development of an International Public Health Genomics Network." *Genetics in Medicine* 8 (7): 451–58.

Chan, Margaret. 2012. "From New Estimates to Better Data." *The Lancet* 380 (9859): 2054.

Chen, Lincoln, and Ling Chen. 2014. "China's Exceptional Health Transitions: Overcoming the Four Horsemen of the Apocalypse." In *Medical Transitions in Twentieth Century China*, edited by Bridie Andrews and Mary Brown Bullock, 17–31. Bloomington: Indiana University Press.

Cutler, David M. 2010. "Where Are the Health Care Entrepreneurs? The Failure of Organizational Innovation in Health Care." *Innovation Policy and the Economy* 11 (1): 1–28.

———. 2013. "Why Medicine Will Be More Like Walmart." *Salon*, September 20. http://www.salon.com/2013/09/20/why_medicine_will_be_more_like_walmart_newscred/. Accessed May 12, 2015.

Gilmour, Stuart, Yi Liao, Ver Bilano, and Kenji Shibuya. 2014. "Burden of Disease in Japan: Using National and Subnational Data to Inform Local Health Policy." *Journal of Preventive Medicine and Public Health* [*Yebang Uihakhoe Chi*] 47 (3): 136–43.

Hashimoto, Hideki, Naoki Ikegami, Kenji Shibuya, Nobuyuki Izumida, Haruko Noguchi, Hideo Yasunaga, Hiroaki Miyata, et al. 2011. "Cost Containment and Quality of Care in Japan: Is There a Trade-Off?" *The Lancet* 378 (9797): 1174–82.

Horton, Richard. 2010. "A New Epoch for Health Professionals' Education." *The Lancet* 376 (9756): 1875–77.

———. 2012. "GBD 2010: Understanding Disease, Injury, and Risk." *The Lancet* 380 (9859): 2053–54.

Ikeda, Nayu, Eiko Saito, Naoki Kondo, Manami Inoue, Shunya Ikeda, Toshihiko Satoh, Koji Wada, Andrew Stickley, et al. 2011. "What Has Made the Population of Japan Healthy?" *The Lancet* 378 (9796): 1094–105.

Ikeda, Nayu, Manami Inoue, Hiroyasu Iso, Shunya Ikeda, Toshihiko Satoh, Mitsuhiko Noda, Tetsuya Mizoue, et al. 2012. "Adult Mortality Attributable to Preventable Risk Factors for Non-Communicable Diseases and Injuries in Japan: A Comparative Risk Assessment." *PLoS Medicine* 9 (1): e1001160.

Ikegami, Naoki, Byung-Kwang Yoo, Hideki Hashimoto, Masatoshi Matsumoto, Hiroya Ogata, Akira Babazono, Ryo Watanabe, et al. 2011. "Japanese Universal Health Coverage: Evolution, Achievements, and Challenges." *The Lancet* 378 (9796): 1106–15.

Institute for Health Metrics and Evaluation. 2012. "About GBD." Last accessed March 17, 2016. http://www.healthdata.org/gbd/about.

———. 2013. *The Global Burden of Disease: Generating Evidence, Guiding Policy*. Seattle, WA: Institute for Health Metrics and Evaluation.

Jason, Hilliard, and Andrew Douglas. 2015. "Are the Conditions Right for a 21st-Century Medical School?" *The Lancet* 385 (9969): 672–73.

Khang, Young-Ho. 2013. "Burden of Noncommunicable Diseases and National Strategies to Control Them in Korea." *Journal of Preventive Medicine and Public Health* 46 (4): 155–64.

Kim, Jim Yong. 2012. "Data for Better Health—and to Help End Poverty." *The Lancet* 380 (9859): 2055.

The Lancet Editors. 2013. "Towards Better Health for People in China." *The Lancet* 381 (9882): 1959.

Lim, Stephen S., Theo Vos, Abraham D. Flaxman, Goodarz Danaei, Kenji Shibuya, Heather Adair-Rohani, Mohammad A. AlMazroa, et al. 2012. "A Comparative Risk Assessment of Burden of Disease and Injury Attributable to 67 Risk Factors and Risk Factor Clusters in 21 Regions, 1990-2010: A Systematic Analysis for the Global Burden of Disease Study 2010." *The Lancet* 380 (9859): 2224-60.

Lozano, Rafael, Mohsen Naghavi, Kyle Foreman, Stephen Lim, Kenji Shibuya, Victor Aboyans, Jerry Abraham, et al. 2012. "Global and Regional Mortality from 235 Causes of Death for 20 Age Groups in 1990 and 2010: A Systematic Analysis for the Global Burden of Disease Study 2010." *The Lancet* 380 (9859): 2095-128.

Marmot, Michael. 2005. "Social Determinants of Health Inequalities." *The Lancet* 365 (9464): 1099-104.

———. 2013. "Universal Health Coverage and Social Determinants of Health." *The Lancet* 382 (9900): 1227-28.

Miyata, Hiroaki, Satoshi Ezoe, Manami Hori, Machiko Inoue, Kazumasa Oguro, Toshihisa Okamoto, Kensuke Onishi, et al. 2015. "Japan's Vision for Health Care in 2035." *The Lancet* 385 (9987): 2549-50.

Murray, Christopher J. L. 2011. "Why is Japanese Life Expectancy So High?" *The Lancet* 378 (9797): 1124-25.

Murray, Christopher J. L., Majid Ezzati, Abraham D. Flaxman, Stephen Lim, Rafael Lozano, Catherine Michaud, Mohsen Naghavi, Joshua A. Salomon, Kenji Shibuya, Theo Vos, Daniel Wikler, and Alan D Lopez. 2012. "GBD 2010: Design, Definitions, and Metrics." *The Lancet* 380 (9859): 2063-66.

Murray, Chistopher, Theo Vos, Rafael Lozano, Mohsen Naghavi, Abraham D. Flaxman, Catherine Michaud, Majid Ezzati, et al. 2012. "Disability-Adjusted Life Years (DALYs) for 291 Diseases and Injuries in 21 Regions, 1990-2010: A Systematic Analysis for the Global Burden of Disease Study 2010." *The Lancet* 380 (9859): 2197-223.

Murray, Chistopher, and Alan D. Lopez. 2013. "Measuring the Global Burden of Disease." *New England Journal of Medicine* 369 (5): 448-57.

Ng, Marie, Tom Fleming, Margaret Robinson, Blake Thomson, Nicholas Graetz, Christopher Margono, Erin C. Mullany, et al. 2014. "Global, Regional, and National Prevalence of Overweight and Obesity in Children and Adults During 1980-2013: A Systematic Analysis for the Global Burden of Disease Study 2013." *The Lancet* 384 (9945): 766-81.

Porter, Michael E., and Elizabeth Olmsted Teisberg. 2006. *Redefining Health Care: Creating Value-Based Competition on Results*. Boston: Harvard Business School Press.

Roth, Gregory A., Stephan D. Fihn, Ali H. Mokdad, Wichai Aekplakorn, Toshihiko Hasegawa, and Stephen S. Lim. 2011. "High Total Serum Cholesterol, Medication Coverage and Therapeutic Control: An Analysis of National Health Examination Survey Data from Eight Countries." *Bulletin of the World Health Organization* 89 (2): 92-101.

Sen, Amartya. 1995. "Mortality as an Indicator of Economic Success and Failure." *UNICEF*. Last accessed May 12, 2015. https://www.unicef-irc.org/publications/pdf/il_mortality.pdf.

Shibuya, Kenji. 2011. *Comprehensive Assessment of the Health System in Japan*. Tokyo: Ministry of Health Labour and Welfare.

Shibuya, Kenji, Hideki Hashimoto, Naoki Ikegami, Akihiro Nishi, Tetsuya Tanimoto, Hiroaki Miyata, Keizo Takemi, et al. 2011. "Future of Japan's System of Good Health at Low Cost with Equity: Beyond Universal Coverage." *The Lancet* 378 (9798): 1265-73.

Tachiya H. 2011. "*Riyakā* [Demountables]." Soma City Mayor's Blog. Last accessed January 10, 2015. http://www.city.soma.fukushima.jp/0311_jishin/melma/20110808_melma.html.

United Nations Population Division. 2012. *World Population Prospects: The 2012 Revision Population Database*. New York: United Nations Population Division.

Wagstaff, Adam. 2005. "Health Systems in East Asia: What Can Developing Countries Learn from Japan and the Asian Tigers?" Policy Research Working Paper 3790. Washington, DC: World Bank Publications.

Woodward, David, Nick Drager, Robert Beaglehole, and Debra Lipson. 2001. "Globalization and Health: A Framework for Analysis and Action." *Bulletin of the World Health Organization* 79 (9): 875–81.

World Health Organization. 1986. "The Ottawa Charter for Health Promotion: First International Conference on Health Promotion, Ottawa, 21 November 1986." Last accessed January 10, 2015. http://www.who.int/healthpromotion/conferences/previous/ottawa/en/.

———. 2010. *A Conceptual Framework for Action on the Social Determinants of Health*. Geneva: World Health Organization.

Yang, Gonghuan, Yu Wang, Yixin Zeng, George F. Gao, Xiaofeng Liang, Maigeng Zhou, Xia Wan, Shicheng Yu, et al. 2013. "Rapid Health Transition in China, 1990–2010: Findings from the Global Burden of Disease Study 2010." *The Lancet* 381 (9882): 1987–2015.

Yang, Seungmi, Young-Ho Khang, Sam Harper, George Davey Smith, David A. Leon, and John Lynch. 2010. "Understanding the Rapid Increase in Life Expectancy in South Korea." *American Journal of Public Health* 100 (5): 896–903.

Yang, Seungmi, Young-Ho Khang, Heeran Chun, Sam Harper, and John Lynch. 2012. "The Changing Gender Differences in Life Expectancy in Korea 1970–2005." *Social Science & Medicine* 75 (7): 1280–87.

Contributors

Mary Brown Bullock has served as Executive Vice Chancellor of Duke Kunshan University, President of Agnes Scott College, and Chair of the China Medical Board. She is currently Vice Chair of the Asia Foundation, a Director of the Henry Luce Foundation and the National Committee on US-China Relations, a Trustee of Agnes Scott College, and a member of the Council of Foreign Relations. Most recently, she has authored *The Oil Prince's Legacy: Rockefeller Philanthropy in China* (Stanford University Press, 2011) and coedited *Medical Transitions in Twentieth Century China* (Indiana University Press, 2014).

Jesse B. Bump is Lecturer on Global Health Policy in the Department of Global Health and Population at the Harvard T. H. Chan School of Public Health. His research interests include the political economy of health and the historical development of health systems. He has authored numerous articles in these areas, including "The Long Road to Universal Health Coverage: Historical Analysis of Early Decisions in Germany, the United Kingdom, and the United States," published in *Health Systems & Reform*.

Lincoln C. Chen is President of the China Medical Board, an independent American foundation endowed by the Rockefeller family for advancing health in China and Asia by strengthening medical education, research, and policies. He was the founding director of the Harvard Global Equity Initiative, Taro Takemi Professor of International Health at the Harvard T. H. Chan School of Public Health, and Director of the Harvard Center for Population and Development Studies. Dr. Chen is chair of the Board of BRAC USA and formerly chaired the Board of CARE/USA.

Yu-Ting Chiu is Research Assistant at the National Taiwan University College of Medicine, Department of Medical Education and Bioethics. She earned an MEd in educational policy and administration from National Taiwan Normal University. Some of her notable coauthored publications include "Effects of Hospital Accreditation on Medical Education: A National Qualitative Study" in *Academic Medicine* and "A Cross-Cultural Study of Students' Approaches to Professional Dilemmas: Sticks or Ripples" in *Medical Education*.

Paul J. Cruickshank is Research Associate at the Institute for Science, Technology, and Society at Tsinghua University. His research interests include the history of global health and the political economy of medical technologies. He lives and works in Beijing, China.

Stuart Gilmour is Associate Professor in the Department of Global Health Policy at the University of Tokyo. He has published research and opinions on global health policy in journals such as *The Lancet*, *BMJ*, and *The Journal of the American Medical Association* and is a Global Burden of Disease Study 2015 collaborator.

Ming-Jung Ho is Professor in the Graduate Institute Department of Medical Education and Bioethics, Vice Chairman of the School of Medicine, and Assistant Dean for International Affairs at National Taiwan University College of Medicine. She earned a BA in biological anthropology from Harvard University, an MD from University of Pennsylvania, and an MPhil in ethnology and museum ethnography from Oxford University, where she also received a DPhil in social anthropology. Dr. Ho's teaching and academic interest lies in the application of anthropology to medical education, and she has published articles in leading international journals.

Yang Ke is Executive Vice President of Peking University and a Foreign Associate at the National Academy of Medicine (formerly the Institute of Medicine). She was Executive Vice President of Peking University Health Science Center (2004–2016).

Gabriel M. Leung is Dean of Medicine and Chair Professor of Public Health Medicine at the University of Hong Kong. Previously, he was Hong Kong's Under Secretary for Food and Health, after which he became Director of the Chief Executive's Office in the government.

OkRyun Moon is Professor Emeritus at Seoul National University. His publications include *Distributive Justice of Health Services* and *Sixty Years of Community Health Service in Korea* (Korea Human Resource Development Institute, 2013).

Kenichi Ohmi is Senior Research Officer at the National Institute of Public Health, Department of Health Promotion, in Japan. Dr. Ohmi is also affiliated with the Japanese Society of Public Health and the Japanese Society for the History of Medicine. His publications include "Estimation of the Excess Death Associated with Influenza Pandemics and Epidemics in Japan After World War II: Relation with Pandemics and the Vaccination System" and "The Vital Statistics in Japan Before World War II—The Transition of the Viewpoint About Nation in the Listing in Vital Statistics Reports," both in *Nihon Koshu Eisei Zasshi* [*Japanese Journal of Public Health*].

N. G. (Niv) Patil is Honorary Clinical Professor in the Department of Surgery and Senior Adviser to the Bau Institute of Medical and Health Sciences Education (BIMHSE) at the University of Hong Kong.

Michael R. Reich is Taro Takemi Professor of International Health Policy at the Harvard T. H. Chan School of Public Health. He received his PhD in political science from Yale University in 1981 and has been a member of the Harvard faculty since 1983. Dr. Reich has longstanding interests in the political economy of health reform, pharmaceutical policy, and Japanese health policy. He is author (with M. J. Roberts, W. Hsiao, and P. Berman) of *Getting Health Reform Right: A Guide to Improving Performance and Equity* (Oxford University Press, 2004) and (with L. J. Frost) *Access: How Do Good Health Technologies Get to Poor People in Poor Countries?* (Frost, Harvard University Press, 2008) and is coeditor in chief of a new journal called *Health Systems & Reform*.

Jennifer Ryan is Chief Operations Officer at the China Medical Board's Equity Initiative program in Southeast Asia. Her degree is from Harvard University's Department of Regional Studies East Asia, where her research focused on the cultural history of medicine in China and the West. Recently she coedited *Philanthropy for Health in China* (Indiana University Press, 2014).

Kevin Shaw worked as Research Assistant in the Department of Medical Education and Bioethics at the National Taiwan University College of Medicine, where he cowrote several papers, including "Equal, Global, Local: Discourses in Taiwan's International Medical Graduate Debate." As a Fulbright fellow, he conducted field research in China in partnership with Chengdu Tongle Health Counseling and Service Center. He is the recipient of a Blakemore Freeman Fellowship for advanced Chinese language studies.

Kenji Shibuya is Professor and Chair of Global Health Policy at the University of Tokyo's Graduate School of Medicine and President of the Japan Institute for Global Health. He has published widely on mortality, causes of death, burden of disease, risk factors, cost-effectiveness, priority setting, health system performance assessment, and health diplomacy. He spearheaded the future strategic directions of the Japanese global health policy agenda after the Hokkaido Toyako G8 Summit in 2008, led *The Lancet*'s series on Japan (published in 2011 in an effort to jumpstart debates on Japanese domestic and global health policy reform), and chaired the landmark Advisory Panel on Health Care 2035 for the Minister of Health, Labour, and Welfare this year.

Julie Shih earned a BS in Health, Science, Society, and Policy and was Research Assistant at the National Taiwan University College of Medicine, Department of Medical Education and Bioethics. She coauthored publications such as "A Comparative Study of Professional and Interprofessional Values between Health Professional Associations" in *The Journal of Interprofessional Care*.

Keizo Takemi is a member of the House of Councillors of the Japanese parliament, or Diet, where he belongs to the Liberal Democratic Party and served in the first Abe administration's cabinet as Senior Vice Minister for Health, Labour, and Welfare. He has been a Senior Fellow with the Japan Center for International Exchange (JCIE) since 2007, and was a research fellow at the Harvard School of Public Health from November 2007 to June 2009. He is also a visiting professor at a number of universities around the country, including Keio University and Nagasaki University. In March 2016, he was appointed to the UN High Level Commission on Health Employment and Economic Growth.

Yusuke Tsugawa is Research Associate in the Department of Health Policy and Management, Harvard T. H. Chan School of Public Health. After practicing as a clinician for several years in Japan, he completed a Harvard-wide general medicine research fellowship at Beth Israel Deaconess Medical Center/Harvard Medical School and worked for the World Bank Group as a Health Specialist. He received his MD from Tohoku University School of Medicine (Japan), MPH from Harvard School of Public Health, and PhD health policy in health policy from Harvard University.

Bong-Min Yang, PhD, is Professor of Health Economics at the Seoul National University, South Korea, where he served as Dean. He also served as President of the Korea Health Economic Association and of the Korea Association of Health Technology Assessment. He currently is

Coeditor in Chief of *Value in Health Regional Issues* and Associate Editor of *Journal of Comparative Effectiveness Research*.

Daqing Zhang is Professor of History of Medicine and Director of the Institute of Medical Humanities at Peking University, as well as Director of the Commission for the History of Medicine, Chinese Society for the History of Science and Technology. His research interests include the cultural and social history of medicine in nineteenth- and twentieth-century China, comparative history, and medical cultures since the late nineteenth century. His recent books include *A History of Medicine* (Peking University Press, 2007) and *An Introduction to Medical Humanities* (Science Press, 2013), both in Chinese.

Index

NOTE: Page numbers in italics indicate illustrations in the text.

Accreditation Board of Medical Education (ABME), Korea, 166
Accreditation Council for Graduate Medical Education (ACGME), 97
accreditation systems: Hong Kong, 121–122, 123, 124; Japan, 143; Korea, 166, 173–174; medical education, 91–92, 97–98; shared challenges in greater China, 104, 124
acupuncture, 8
Adams, Walter, 119
aging of population, 188–189, 200–204
Alice Memorial Hospital (Hong Kong), 114
Allen, Horace N., 159–160
American Bureau for Medical Aid to China, 89
Anatomische Tabellen (Kulmus), 131
assistant doctors, 64
Association of Korean Medicine, 16
Association of Southeast Asian Nations (ASEAN), 124
Avison, Oliver R., 160

Bane Report (Surgeon General's Consultant Group on Medical Education, 1959), 45
barefoot doctors, 16–17, 23
Beijing Medical College, 65
Bell, Adam Schall von, 158
Bell, John, 114
Belz, Erwin von, 152
Berry, George Packer, 43
Bill and Melinda Gates Foundation, 200
biomedical research training, 50
Black, Davidson, 23
Boguyeogwan Hospital (Korea), 160
Boji Medical School (Hong Kong), 115
Bretton Woods institutions, 46, 51
British medical education: adoption of model in Hong Kong, 9, 113, 122; characteristics, 10
Bullock, Mary Brown, 10–11
Bump, Jesse B., 11
burden of disease: about, 187; declines in rapid aging and mortality, 188–189; disease estimation and policy development, 199–200; health policy in East Asia and, 200–205; health transitions, 189–193; population health profiles, 200–201; risk factors, 190, 199. *See also* Global Burden of Disease (GBD) study

Cambodia: CMB support for, 32
Cantlie, James, 114
Carnegie Foundation for the Advancement of Teaching, 39
Case Western Reserve University, 42, 43
Chalmers, John, 114
Chang Gung School of Medicine (Taiwan), 90
Chen, C. C., 23
Chen, Lincoln, 34
Chen Zhu, 77
China
 barefoot doctors, 16–17, 23
 burden of disease: analysis and policy development, 195; disability-adjusted life years, 189, *190*; epidemiologic transitions, 189, 190, *197*; life expectancy and mortality changes since World War II, 189; risk factors, 190, 199
 China Medical Board: grants and endowment funding, 32–33; return to China (1981), 32–34, 74–75; withdrawal from mainland (1951), 24
 Chinese Civil War (1927–1949), 62
 Great Leap Forward, 69
 health indicators and medical education, 5–8, *6*
 medical education since 1949 (PRC), 11–12, 61–81; adoption of international educational standards, 76–77; assistant doctors (medical assistants), 64–65; clinical specialties training, 63–64; Cultural Revolution disruptions, 9, 15, 70–72, 80; development period (1993–), 75–77; differing types of, 16–17, 62–64, 81n2; expansion of medical schools, 69; health care management training, 81n1; human resource allocation problems, 78–79; Mao's criticism of, 69–70;

215

China (*continued*)
  maternal and children's health care workers, 64–65; medical elitism vs. populism in, 80–81; medical manpower shortages, 62–63; merger of Western and Chinese medical colleges, 71–72, 72, 80; midwives and nurses, 64; National College Entrance Examination (*gaokao*), 73; Nationalist medical schools, 62; neglect of humanities and social sciences, 77, 78; new education system (1949–1952), 62–65; politics affecting, 79–80; reconstruction period (1977–1993), 73–75; reforms in (1952–1965), 65, 68–70; reforms since 1993, 75–77; regional distribution of medical training, 73; reorganization of medical colleges, 65, 66–67, 68; rural health care workers as priority, 77; science and technology training priorities, 74; Soviet model of health care, 9, 65, 79–80, 113; tradition vs. modernity in, 80; traditional Chinese medicine incorporated into, 68–69; training of minority health professionals, 73; transition to Anglo-American health care model, 10; visual teaching methods, 64
  Regulation of Universities (1912), 61
  Republic of China: establishment of (1912), 9; Kuomintang relocation to Taiwan, 88 (*See also* Taiwan)
  Tiananmen Square protests, 33
China Medical Board (CMB)
  challenges for 21st century, 34–35
  institutional history of, 21–36; centenary celebration, 3, 34; Cultural Revolution impact on programs, 15–16; as direct operating foundation, 34; extension of programs to East and Southeast Asia, 24–32; PUMC era, 22–24; return to mainland China (1981), 32–34, 74–75; Rockefeller Foundation and establishment of, 22, 46; withdrawal from China (1951), 24
  medical education support in East Asia, 10–11, 21–22; medical university grants (1951–2000), 25, *25*, 35–36; South Korea, 165, 168–170, *170*; Taiwan, 89
  program funding by era: in 1960s, 29; in 1970s, 30–32; since 2007, 34, 74
  types of support: block grants, 30; endowment grants, 31; fellowship program (1951–1973), 26, *27*, 30; grant funding after 1981, 32–33; laboratory equipment and supplies, 28;

medical education conferences, 29; medical libraries, 27–28; post-war construction and building renovation grants, 28; Program of Higher Nursing Education Development (POHNED), 33; project funding (venture capital), 33; regional development, 30, 32–33; telecommunications and telemedicine grants, 33–34; visiting professorships, 26–27
China Medical College (Taiwan), 90
China Medical Commission, Rockefeller Foundation, 22–23
China Medical University, 16, 63
Chinese Civil War (1927–1949), 62
Chinese Imperial Maritime Customs Service, 85
Chinese medicine. *See* traditional Chinese medicine (TCM)
Chinese Undergraduate Medical Education Standards, 77
Chinese University of Hong Kong, 120–121
cholera research program (NIH), 48–49
Chonnam University Medical College, 168
Christian Hospital (Changhu), 85
Chung Shan Medical and Dental College, 90
Clementi, Cecil, 115–116
clinical performance examinations, 166, 172
clinical skills tests, 167
clinical training: China, 63–64; Hong Kong, 116; Japan, 144, 146; South Korea, 172; Taiwan, 99–100, 103; United States, 44–45, 52
CMB. *See* China Medical Board (CMB)
colonialism: impact on medical education, 14–15
Communist Party of China (CPC): medical schools under, 62
Confucius, 152
continuing medical education: South Korea, 173–174; Taiwan, 91
Council on Medical Education (Japan), 142
Cox, Christopher, 118
Creech-Jones, Arthur, 118
Cruickshank, Paul J., 11
Cultural Revolution (1966–1976): "barefoot doctors" movement, 16–17; impact on CMB programs, 15–16; medical curriculum changes, 71; medical education and, 9, 15, 70–72, 80
cultural values and medical education, 104–105
Curriculum Guide for Chinese Medical Universities and Colleges (1998), 76

Daegu Medical College, 164
Daehan Hospital/Medical School (Korea), 162, 163
Daewongun (Korean regent), 158

Davison, Wilbert C., 89
Deng Xiaoping, 74, 113
Dongdaemun Hospital (Lillian Harris Memorial Hospital for Children), 161
Dongje School (Korea), 161–162

East Asia: future of health policy in, 200–205; map of, 7. *See also* medical education in East Asia
East-West Alliance, 125, 127n2
Economic Developing Cooperation Fund (EDCF), 176
Edinburgh Declaration, World Federation for Medical Education (1988), 75
Eulsa Treaty (1905), 162
Ewha Medical College, 168

faculty development: Taiwan medical schools, 97
Flexner, Abraham, 39
Flexner Report (*Medical Education in the United States and Canada*, 1910): focus on scientific research and practice, 38, 39; influence on medical education, 5, 10, 11; Japanese medical education reforms and, 144; on quality of medical profession, 45; reform of Flexnerian educational model, 42–44
Fogarty, John E., 40
Fogarty International Center (FIC), 50
Foulk, G. C., 159
Frenk, Julio, 125, 126
Fu Jen Catholic University College of Medicine, 90

Gachon College of Medical Science, 164
Gault, N. J., 169
GBD. *See* Global Burden of Disease (GBD) study
General Headquarters/Supreme Commander for the Allied Powers (GHQ/SCAP), Public Health and Welfare Section, 142
General Medical Training Demonstration Centers (Taiwan), 97
German model of medical education, 9–10, 13, 150–151, *133*
Global Burden of Disease (GBD) study: comparative analysis of risk factors, 190, 199, *198*; disability-adjusted life years, 189, 190, *191–197*; health transitions, 189, 190; history and function of, 188, 205; international health assessment using, 200; partner institutions, 200; process funding and collaboration, 200; sub-national policy development and estimation, 199–200
global health paradigm, 201–203
Global Health Unit, Peking University Health Science Center, 204
Global Leadership Program, University of Tokyo, 204–205
Global Minimum Essential Requirements (GMER), 34
Gojong, King of Korea, 159
Gotu Shimpei, 86
Government Civil Hospital (Queen Mary Hospital), Hong Kong, 113, 117, 119–120
Grant, John B., 23, 24
Grantham, Alexander, 119
Greene, Roger Sherman, 23, 24
Gu Lau Hospital (Tainan), 85
Guidelines for Quality Assurance of Basic Medical Education in the Western Pacific Region (WHO, 2001), 77
Gwangjewon Hospital, 161
Gyeongsung Imperial University Medical College, 163
Gyeongsung Professional Medical School, 163

Hall, William James, 161
Halnan, Keith, 122
Halnan Lecture, 122, 127n1
Hartigan, William, 114
He Cheng, 68
Health Care 2035 (Japan), 202
Health for Peace (1958), 47
health indicators and medical education, 5–8, *6*
health manpower: China, 62–63; East Asia, US, and UK (comparison), *124*; Hong Kong, 123–124; United States, 45
health policy in East Asia: global health paradigm, 201–203
Heron, John W., 160
Hill, Lister, 40
Ho, Ming-Jung, 12
Ho Kai, 114
Hobson, Benjamin, 113, 122
Hong Kong, 112–127
  expansion of welfare state (1970s), 119, 120
  geopolitical events and history of, 112–113
  health indicators and medical education, 5–8, *6*
  health manpower, 123–124
  medical education in: British model for, 9, 10, 12, 113, 122; Chinese University of Hong

Hong Kong (*continued*)
  Kong, 120–121; CMB support for, 25, *25*, 32, 35; Cox Report on, 119, 120; early medical schools, 115; future possibilities for, 122–127; Hong Kong College of Medicine, 12, 112, 114–116; integrative medicine, 126, 127; Japanese occupation impact on, 118–119; Jennings/Logan Report on, 119–120; medical ethics and law courses, 125; MOOCs as challenge for, 125–126; niche areas for expansion, 125; postgraduate training and accreditation, 121–122, 123; postwar decades (1950–1980), 119–120; shortage of health care personnel, 123, *124*; University of Hong Kong Faculty of Medicine, 117–119
  missionaries and introduction of Western medicine, 113–114, 122
  postwar population growth, 119
  service-based economy of, 123
  Sino-British Joint Declaration for repatriation, 121, 122
  traditional Chinese medicine in, 113–114, 126
Hong Kong Academy of Medicine, 12, 121, 122, 124
Hong Kong College of Medicine, 12, 112, 114–116
Houghton, Henry S., 24
Hu Shih, 24
Huang Jiasi, 24, 32

Imperial University (Japan), 136, *138*
Indonesia: CMB support for, 32
infectious disease control, 200, 201
information management and global health, 201–203
informative learning, 126
Institute for International Medical Education (IIME), 34, 77
Institute of Health Metrics and Evaluation, University of Washington, 200
instructional design, 17–18
insurance, health. *See* national health insurance systems
integrative medicine, 126, 127
International Center for Diarrheal Disease Research, Bangladesh, 48
International Cooperation Administration, U.S., 167
International Health Division, Rockefeller Foundation, 45–46
International Health Research Act (U.S., 1960), 46–47
International Standards in Basic Medical Education (WFME, 1999), 77

Inter-University Council for Higher Education in the Colonies, 119
I-Shou University College of Medicine, 90

J. W. Lee Center for Global Medicine, 171
Japan
  burden of disease: analysis and policy development, 195; disability-adjusted life years, 189, *191*; life expectancy and mortality changes since World War II, 188; risk factors, 190, 199, *193*
  health indicators and medical education, 5–8, *6*
  medical education (Edo period–1945), 133–140; Anglo-American model in private medical schools, 138; class division in education and career choice, 133, *133*; CMB funding for, 25, *25*, 32, 35–36; Dutch studies (*Rankagu*), 131–132; German model for, 9, 13, 133–134, *133*; as hierarchical system, 137–138; historical influences on, 133–139; imperial universities, 136, *137*; influence on medical education in Korea and Taiwan, 14–15, 141–143; integration of medical education system (1918), 138; introduction of Western medicine (*Ranpo*), 8, 13, 131–132; licensure of practitioners, 134–138; Medical Law (1874), 137; medical practitioners as artisans, 130; medical professional schools, 135–136; Meiji-era reforms, 137–141; National Examination for Medical Practitioners, 137–138; number of medical schools (1885–1979), *138*; physicians by type of education (1885–1953), 137–138; pre-Meiji Restoration, 131–132; private medical schools, 139, 140, 146; status gap among physicians pre–World War II, 140
  medical education after World War II, 142–154; adoption of American educational model, 9, 10, 143; changes in medical education system, 145–149; Council on Medical Education and, 144; cramming-oriented curriculum, 146, 152–154; curriculum and course changes, 144–145; curriculum hours by type of school (1975–2011), 147, *148*, 149–150, *150*; decline in lectures and liberal arts education, 152–154; desired types of physicians before and after war, 150–151, *150*, *151*; elimination and consolidation of medical professional schools, 142; liberal arts study by type of school (1975–2011), 149–150, *149*; National Examination for Physicians, 143, *144*, 149, 151–154;

new medical schools, 145–146; present state of system, 147–151; public vs. private medical schools, 147; recommended curriculum reforms, 153–154; societal and demographic changes affecting, 145–147
traditional Chinese medicine (*kampo*): Medical Law exclusions for, 167; politics and banning of, 15; practitioners in Edo period, 130–131
universal health insurance system, 145
Japan Society for Oriental Medicine, 16
Japan University Accreditation Association, 144
Japanese Ministry of Health, Labour, and Welfare, 190, 199, 200
Japan–Korea Treaty (1876), 159
Jejungwon Hospital (Seoul), 8, 159–160
Jennings, Ivor, 119
Jeong Yak-yong, 158
Jikei University (Seii-kai), 139
Jones, Mouat, 119
Jordan, Gregory, 114
Joseon Dynasty (Korea), 158
Judson, Harry Pratt, 22

Kanehiro, Takaki, 138
Keijo Women's Medical Professional School (Seoul), 141
Keio University School of Medicine, 139
Keio-gijuku Medical School, 139
KIMEE (Korean Institute of Medical Education and Evaluation), 166, 173
Kipling, Rudyard, 126
KOFIH (Korea Foundation for International Health), 176
Kong Ying-Wa, 115
Korea
burden of disease in South Korea: analysis and policy development, 199; disability-adjusted life years, 189, *192*; epidemiologic transitions, 190; life expectancy and mortality changes since World War II, 189
history of: Eulsa Treaty establishing Japanese protectorate, 162; First Sino-Japanese War, 159; Gapsin Coup (1884), 159; Great Korean Empire (1897–1910), 161; isolationist policies, 158; Japanese-founded hospitals in 19th century, 159; Japan–Korea Treaty (1876), 159; Korean War (1950–1953), 164
medical education, 8, 158–180; Daehan Medical School, 162, 163; following Korean War (*See* South Korea *below*); hospital resources under Japanese colonial rule, 162–163, 163; Japanese influence on, 9, 141–142, 159; medical missionaries and, 159–161; medical school graduates until 1945, 141, *142*; medical schools before and after 1945, 141, *142*, 178–179; missionary hospitals, 160–161; nursing education, 161; post-independence growth of medical schools, 163–164; traditional Chinese medicine, 161–162; transition to Anglo-American model, 10, 13; Uihakgyo introducing Western-style education (1899), 161; Western health care as foreign trade byproduct, 158–159; Western medical schools in Joseon Dynasty, 161
South Korea: accreditation assessment, 173–174; Accreditation Board of Medical Education, 166; American-style medical education in, 164–167; changes in curriculum structure, 171–173; clinical performance examinations, 166, 172; clinical skills tests, 167; CMB grants for medical education, 25, 32, 36, 165, 168–170, *170*; continuing medical education, 173–174; current status of medical education, 170–174; domestic challenges, 175–176; economic expansion and growth of medical colleges, 164, 166; efficiency of health system, 176; exporting Korean health services education model, 174, 175; future prospects for medical education, 174–177; graduate education programs, 171–172; leadership role in international community, 175, 178; mandatory military service, 171–172; medical colleges (1910–2014), *165*; Medical Service Act, 173; Minnesota Project, 167–168; National Health Insurance program, 164; National Teachers Training Center, 165, 171; as official development assistance donor, 171, 176–177; post-war restoration of medical education infrastructure, 165; potential cooperation with North Korea, 177; public health care, 172–173; Seoul National University Medical College (SNUMC), 163, 165; student-centered learning, 166, 172, 173–174
Korea Foundation for International Health (KOFIH), 176
Korea Imperial University, 141
Korea International Cooperation Agency (KOICA), 176
Korean Institute of Medical Education and Evaluation (KIMEE), 166, 173
Korean League of Deans of Medical Colleges, 166
Korean League of Medical Education, 166

Korean Medical Association (KMA), 164, 173
Korean War (1950–1953), 164
Kulmus, Johan Adam, 131
Kuomintang (KMT): medical education under, 88–95; relocation to Taiwan (1945), 88
Kyung-Puk University, 168
Kyushu Imperial University, 140

Landsborough, David, 85
Laos: CMB support for, 32, 33
Lee, C. U., 24
Lee Jong-Wook/Seoul National University Global Project, 174, 205
Leung, Gabriel, 12
Li, Choh-Ming, 120–121
Li Hung-Chang, 115
Li Ka Shing Foundation, 125
licensure of physicians: Japan, 137–138, 144, *134*; Korea, 167; Taiwan, 12, 85, 88–89, 91–92, 95, 98, 101–102; traditional medicine, 92
life expectancy: increase since World War II, 188–189
Liu Shaoqi, 68
Lockhart, William, 113
Logan, Douglas, 119
London Missionary Society, 112–113
Loucks, Harold, 24, 28
Lugard, Frederick, 115

Mackay, George L., 85
Mackay Hospital (Taipei), 85
MacLehose, Murray, 119
Manson, Patrick, 85, 114–115, 116
Mao Zedong: criticism of health care system and medical education, 70; on length of schooling, 69–70; support for Chinese medicine, 68–69
massive open online courses (MOOCs), 125–126
Maxwell, James L., 85
McCoy, Oliver R., 29
McKibbin, George Baldwin, 23
MDGs (Millennium Development Goals), 189
Medical Council of Hong Kong, 116, 121, 123, 125
medical education in East Asia, 3–19; characteristics by country, 7–8; colonialism and, 14–15; common challenges, 16–18, 104–105; competency-based, as shared challenge, 8–9; cross-cutting themes in, 14–18; cultural values and, 104–105; curriculum reforms, 204–205; domestic politics influencing, 15–16; elite vs. popular orientation in different countries, 16–17; Global Leadership Program, University of Tokyo, 204–205; health indicators and, 5–8, *6*; hierarchy of medical institutions, 17; institutional and instructional design, 17–18; international politics influencing, 14–15; linking scientific knowledge and good health, 4; medical missionaries and, 8–9, 102; shared challenges in greater China, 104–105; tradition vs. modernity in, 16; traditional Chinese medicine, 8; Western models in East Asian countries, 8–10. See also *names of specific countries*
"Medical Education in East Asia: Past and Future" (workshop, 2014), 3
Medical Education in the United States and Canada (Flexner, 1910), 39. See also Flexner Report
"Medical Education Revolution" (China), 71
Medical Law (1874), Japan, 137
Medical Missionary Hospital of Hong Kong, 9, 113, 122
medical simulation centers, 166
Medical Training Center (Jejungwong, Korea), 141
medical universities: role and function of, 4
Medicare and Medicaid: US clinical education and, 44–45, 52
Medicine in China (China Medical Commission, Rockefeller Foundation), 22–23
Meerdervoort, J. C. L. Pompe van, 131–132
Millennium Development Goals (MDGs), 189
Min Yeong-Ik, 159
Ministry of Education (MOE), Taiwan, 97
Ministry of Health (MOH), China, 32, 64
Ministry of Health and Welfare, Taiwan, 97
Minnesota Project (Seoul National University Cooperative Project), 167–168, 169–170, 174
missionaries, medical: in Hong Kong, 113–114, 122; in Korea, 159–161; in Taiwan, 85, 102; Western medicine in East Asia and, 8–9, 112–113
Mongolia: CMB support for, 33
MOOCs (massive open online courses), 125–126
Moon, OkRyun, 13
Morrison, Robert, 112
mortality rates: declines since World War II, 188–189
Mutual Security Administration (US), 46, 47, 89
Myanmar: CMB support for, 32, 33

Nagasaki Navy Medical School (*Nagasaki kaigun denshu-sho*), 131
Nanking, Treaty of (1841), 12, 113
National Cheng Kung University School of Medicine (Taiwan), 90

National Committee on Foreign Medical Education and Accreditation (NCFMEA), 91–92
National Defense Medical Center (NDMC, Taiwan), 24, 89, 90
National Examination for Medical Practitioners (Japan), 137–138
National Examination for Physicians (Japan), 145, *134*, 146, 149, 151, 152–154
national health insurance systems: Japan, 145; Korea, 164; Taiwan, 92–93
National Health Research Institute, 92
National Health Services (Taiwan), 86
National Higher Medical Education Conferences (China), 68, 70
National Institutes of Health (NIH): cholera research program, 48–49; as conduit for biomedical research funding, 40–41; conflict between domestic and international research priorities, 49–50, 51, 53; educational goals, 11; fellowships, 48; international projects and research, 47–48, 51–52; Office of International Research, 49; US strategic priorities affecting, 48–49
National Taiwan University College of Medicine (NTUCM), 86, 89, 90
National Teachers Training Center (NTTC), 165, 171
NDMC (National Defense Medical Center), Taiwan, 24, 89, 90
Nepal: CMB support for, 33
New Book of Anatomy (*Kaitai shinsho*, 1774), 131
NIH. *See* National Institutes of Health (NIH)
noncommunicable diseases (NCDs), 198–200, *193*, 205
Norris, Laurie, 31
North Korea: potential South Korean cooperation with, 177
NTTC (National Teachers Training Center), 165, 171
NTUCM (National Taiwan University College of Medicine), 86, 89, 90
nursing education: Korea, 161; Program of Higher Nursing Education Development (CMB), 33; Taiwan, 98–99

Objective Structured Clinical Examination (OSCE), 166
Official Development Assistance (ODA), 171, 176–177
Ohmi, Kenichi, 13
Ongley, Patrick, 26, 30, 31, 32–33, 74
Opium War, Second (1856–1860), 85

Organization for Economic Cooperation and Development (OECD), 164, 171
Outline of Reform and Development of China's Education, 75

Pak Ji-won, 158
Parker, Peter, 113
Parran, Thomas, 41
Patil, N. G. (Niv), 12
PBL. *See* problem-based learning (PBL)
Peabody, Francis Weld, 23
Pearce, Richard, 117
Peiyang (Bei Yang) Medical College (Tianjin), 115
Peking, Treaty of (1860), 85
Peking Union Medical College (PUMC): American foundation support for, 24; barefoot doctor model and, 23; as biomedical research facility, 23–24; CMB relationship with, 15, 22; founding of, 9, 113; impact of Sino-Japanese and Chinese civil wars on, 24; nationalization of, 11, 21, 24; Rockefeller Foundation and, 22, 113
Peking University Health Science Center, Global Health Unit, 205
People's Republic of China (PRC). *See* China
Philippines: CMB support for, 32
Polish medical degrees, 100–101, 103
population in East Asia, 5, 6
postgraduate training: Hong Kong, 121–122, 123; Taiwan, 98
problem-based learning (PBL): CMB support for, 22; limited use in China, 17; as shared challenge for greater China, 104, 118, 125; in South Korea, 173; in Taiwan, 96–97
Program of Higher Nursing Education Development (POHNED), 33
public health: education in Taiwan, 99; South Korea, 172–173
PUMC. *See* Peking Union Medical College (PUMC)
Pusan National University, 168

Qing Dynasty, 84–85
Queen Mary Hospital (Government Civil Hospital), Hong Kong, 113, 117, 119–120

Republic of China. *See* Taiwan
Republic of Korea. *See* South Korea *under* Korea
Rha, Sejin, 169
Ride, Lindsay, 118
Rockefeller, John D. Jr., 23
Rockefeller, John D. III, 22

Rockefeller Foundation: China Medical Commission, 22–23; CMB established as program of, 22, 46; expenditures on international projects, 48; International Health Division programs, 45–46; Peking Union Medical College and, 9; spreading American health care to less developed regions, 46; support for University of Hong Kong Faculty of Medicine, 117
Ross, Ronald, 116
Ryan, Jennifer, 10–11

Sams, Crawford W., 143
Sawyer, Bill, 30, 33
Schwartz, Roy, 33–34
Seii-kai (Jikei University), 139
Sen, Amartya, 188
Seongho Saseol / Mr. Seongho's Discourses on the Minute (Bell), 158
Seoul National University Medical College (SNUMC), 163, 165; Lee Jong-Wook/Seoul National University Global Project, 174, 201; Minnesota Project, 167–168, 169–170, 174
Severance, Louis H., 160
Severance Medical Professional School (Korea), 141
Shannon, James, 40, 48
Sherwood, Rosetta, 161
Shibasaburo, Kitasato, 139
Shibuya, Kenji, 13
Singapore: CMB support for, 32
Sino-Japanese War, First (1894–1895), 85, 159
Sloss, Duncan, 118–119
SNUMC. *See* Seoul National University Medical College (SNUMC)
South Korea. *See under* Korea
Southeast Asia Treaty Organization (SEATO), 48
Soviet health care model: adoption in China, 9, 113; characteristics, 10; medical education and, 65, 79–80
Specht, Heinz, 50
Standards for Establishing Medical Schools (1968), Japan, 146
Stanford University, 42, 43
State Administration of Traditional Chinese Medicine, 16
Stewart, Frederick, 114
Sudo Medical College, 168
Sun Yat-Sen, 23, 115

Sun Yat-Sen University, Zhongshan School of Medicine, 115
Surgeon General's Consultant Group on Medical Education (Bane Report, 1959), 45

Tagore, Rabindranath, 178
Taihoku Imperial University (Taipei), 141
Taipei Medical College, 90
Taipei Medical University, 89
Taiwan
  challenges for medical education: clinical competence, 99–100; current reforms, 101–102; global standards vs. local needs, 103; inflexibility of educational system, 100; politics of international education, 100–101, 103; professional prospects, 102–103; shared with greater China, 104–105; subsidizing costs for clinical teaching, 103
  Council for Economic Planning and Development, 92
  Department of Health, 91
  expatriate medical community, 102
  health indicators and medical education, 5–8, 6
  health system data, comparative, 105–106
  history of: colonization by Dutch and Spanish (17th century), 84; immigrants and dominance of traditional Chinese medicine, 84; indigenous practitioners in colonial period, 84; introduction of Western medicine, 8, 84–85; Japanese colonialism, 85–88, 102; medical and public health infrastructure under Japanese rule, 86–87; Qing Dynasty rule, 84–85
  medical education, 84–106; accreditation and quality assurance, 91–92, 97–98; CMB support for, 25, 32, 36; continuing education, 91; current state of, 95–99; faculty development, 97; as hybrid system, 102–103; internal factors and actors, 93–95, 94; Japanese colonialism and, 141–142; KMT government and, 88–95; legitimizing colonial rule, 86–87; licensure of physicians, 12, 85, 88–89, 91–92, 95, 98, 101–102; medical colleges and universities, 105; as national mission, 91; Postgraduate General Medical Training program, 92; postgraduate training, 98; post-World War II influences on, 9, 93–95; private medical schools, 90–91; student selection, 95–96; Taiwan Education Law, 86; teaching hospitals, 93, 97;

traditional Chinese medicine, 84, 87, 92; transition from Japanese to American education model, 90; US aid and influence, 89–90, 102; as vehicle for modernization, 12, 84, 86
missionary medicine, 85, 102
National Health Insurance (NHI), 92–93
nursing education, 98–99
public health education, 99
Republic of China: establishment on mainland (1912), 9; KMT relocation from mainland (1945), 88; negative impact of KMT transfer on physician training and licensure, 88–89
Taiwan Association of Medical Education (TAME), 97
Taiwan Imperial University, 141
Taiwan Medical Accreditation Council (TMAC), 92, 97–98
Taiwanese Doctors Association, 88
Takada Eisaku, 158
TCM. *See* traditional Chinese medicine (TCM)
teaching hospitals: burden of disease on, 45; clinical practice revenues in, 44–45; Hong Kong, 117; Korea, 160, 161; Taiwan, 93, 97; United States, 44
Thailand: CMB support for, 32
Tiananmen Square protests (1989), 33
Tianjin, Treaty of (1858), 85
Tibet Medical College, 33
TMAC (Taiwan Medical Accreditation Council), 92
Todd, David, 122
Tokyo Medical School, 132, 137
Tokyo Women's Medical School, 140
Tomoyasu, Sagara, 132
traditional Chinese medicine (TCM): coexistence with Western medicine, 16; colleges of, 69; Communist government support for, 68–69; domestic politics and banning of, 15; in Hong Kong, 113–114, 126; incorporation into higher medical education, 68–69, 71–72; integrative medicine model, 126; in Korea, 161–162; medicinal treatments and theories, 8; merger of Western and Chinese medical colleges during Cultural Revolution, 71–72, 72, 80; in Taiwan, 84, 87, 92
Treaty of Nanking (1841), 12, 113
Treaty of Peking (1860), 85
Treaty of Tianjin (1858), 85
Tu Tsung-ming, 90

Tung Wah Hospital (Hong Kong), 113–114
Tzu Chi University College of Medicine, 90

UCLA (University of California, Los Angeles), 42, 43
Union Medical College (Beijing), 23
United States
    development assistance activities during Cold War, 47, 52
    federal funding for biomedical research, 40–42
    foreign policy and international health initiatives, 45–52, 53, 55n18
    International Cooperation Administration, 167
    medical education in, 38–55; biomedical research, 43, 50–51; characteristics, 10; clinical education, 44–45, 52; core science courses with electives model, 42–44; evolution of, 11; federal funding for research shaping curriculum, 39–42, 52; Flexner Report and transformation of, 5, 10, 11, 38, 39; health manpower and, 45; international influence of, 38–39; medical schools as research institutions, 41; Medicare/Medicaid impacts on, 44–45, 52; overview, 38–39; reform of Flexnerian model, 42–44; trends in mid-20th century, 38
    Mutual Security Administration, 46
    post-World War II research and educational developments, 39–45, 52
    public support for government-sponsored research, 39–40
    research support and balance-of-payments problems, 51–52, 54. *See also* National Institutes of Health (NIH)
University of California, Los Angeles (UCLA), 42, 43
University of Hong Kong Faculty of Medicine: changed mission following World War II, 118–119; CMB endowment grant to, 31; historical importance of, 112; Hong Kong College of Medicine transition, 116; Japanese occupation effects on, 118–119; medical humanities curriculum, 125; post-war infrastructure improvements, 120; pre-World War II growth, 117–118; School of Chinese Medicine, 16
University of Minnesota, 167
University of Tokyo, Global Leadership Program, 204–205
University of Tsukuba, 147

University of Washington, Institute of Health Metrics and Evaluation, 200
US Agency for International Development (US-AID), 47

Vietnam: CMB support for, 29, 32, 33
Vinton, C. C., 160
Virchow, Rudolf, 112

Wang Bin, 63
Willis, William, 140
World Federation for Medical Education (WFME): Edinburgh Declaration (1988), 75; International Standards in Basic Medical Education (1999), 77
World Health Organization (WHO): Global Burden of Disease study and, 200; Guidelines for Quality Assurance of Basic Medical Education in the Western Pacific Region (2001), 77
Wu Jieping, 24, 32

Yang Ming School of Medicine (Taipei), 90
Yayoi, Yoshioka, 140
Yi Gyu-gyeong, 158
Yi-Ik (1681–1763), 158
Yonsei University: CMB support for, 28, 31
Yonsei University Medical College, 168, 169
Yoshio, Kusama, 142
Young, William, 114
Yu Yiti, 62–63

Zhang Daqing, 11
Zhou Enlai, 68, 72